Focus on Cancer

Springer

London
Berlin
Heidelberg
New York
Barcelona
Budapest
Hong Kong
Milan
Paris
Santa Clara
Singapore
Tokyo

Robert Dunlop

Cancer: Palliative Care

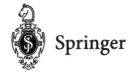 Springer

Robert Dunlop
St Christopher's Hospice
51-59 Lawrie Park Road
Sydenham
London SE26 6DZ, UK

ISBN 3-540-19974-8 Springer-Verlag Berlin Heidelberg New York

British Library Cataloguing in Publication Data
Dunlop, Robert
 Cancer : palliative care.   -   (Focus on cancer)
 1.Cancer - Palliative treatment
 I.Title
 616.9'94'06
 ISBN 3540199748

Library of Congress Cataloging-in-Publication Data
Dunlop, Robert, 1956-
 Cancer : palliative care / Robert Dunlop.
    p.   cm. - - (Focus on cancer)
 Includes bibliographical references and index.
 ISBN 3-540-19974-8 (pbk. : alk. paper)
 1. Cancer- -Palliative treatment.   I. Title.   II. Series.
 [DNLM: 1. Neoplasms- -therapy.   2. Palliative Care- -methods.
 3. Pain, intractable- -therapy.   QZ 266 D922c 1998]
 RC271.P33D86   1998
 616.99'406- -dc21
 DNLM/DLC   97-36628
 for Library of Congress   CIP

Typeset by Richard Powell Editorial and Production Services, Basingstoke, Hants RG22 4TX
Printed and bound at the Athenæum Press Ltd., Gateshead, Tyne and Wear
28/3830-543210 Printed on acid-free paper

Contents

Foreword

Hospice and palliative care are now recognised internationally, but far too many patients still fail to receive its benefits. Much of the groundwork has been researched, developed and demonstrated, but all countries need access to the publications which will spread the knowledge.

Every patient needs appropriate and individualised treatment throughout the course of illness. Not all can be cured and all will eventually die. How that happens is not only important for their dignity as individuals but also as members of a family network. A life ended with much unfinished business or uncontrolled suffering has not been met with due respect and does not leave good memories. To accept that life is ending can give value, freedom and hope. Openness and the respectful sharing of bad news can lead to creativity and the healing of relationships. Those of us who have travelled alongside many people at the end of their lifes' journeys have seen not merely endurance and courage, but much growth through loss.

All this calls for great competence in the analysis and relief of the various forms of suffering that make up the Total Pain of a terminal illness. Much evidence-based therapy is available and is presented in this compassionate, practical and challenging book. 'Efficiency is very comforting', said one family member. It is indeed comforting, both to the patient, family members and to the staff team caring for them. The past decades have seen much learning of psychological, social and spiritual, as well as physical, needs. This book, the fruit of years of experience, brings understanding and help to all those who set out to give the best, most appropriate and personal care to those facing the end of life. There is medical challenge, reward and personal hope in the possibilities of the human being whose final needs and potential demand our attention.

Dame Cicely Saunders, OM, DBE, FRCP
Chairman, St. Christopher's Hospice, London

Preface

Despite major advances in diagnosis and treatment, cancer remains a leading cause of death. Traditionally, people were told 'nothing more can be done' when anti-cancer treatments were exhausted or not possible. This left patients and families feeling abandoned, facing the worst part of the illness alone. Palliative care offers hope and support to patients with advanced, incurable cancer, and to their families. It has become a recognised specialty with a rapidly expanding knowledge base that has spread worldwide.

This book provides an introduction to palliative care as part of the Springer Focus on Cancer series. It offers a broad overview of the specialty, complementing the other books in the series on anti-cancer treatments and on psychological support for cancer patients. It has been written for health professionals from all disciplines, particularly doctors and nurses who work with cancer patients but have little or no experience of palliative care.

The opening chapter presents an overview of palliative care and its development. Throughout history, the care of the dying has been neglected. A review of the reasons for this emphasises the important issues for the future, such as the desire of patients for cure and the difficulties that health professionals have with death and dying. The principles of palliative care are outlined, including patient and family care, multi-disciplinary teamwork and bereavement support.

The next chapters describe how to control the myriad of symptoms of cancer including pain, nausea, vomiting and breathlessness. Useful therapies are highlighted, as well as the potential psychological attributions which affect patients and families just as much as the physical symptoms. This leads into the chapter on psycho-social care and suffering. A chapter is devoted to the practicalities of team working which is so essential to dealing with the needs of cancer patients and families.

Some readers will be interested in a career in palliative care. There is a chapter which describes the variety of settings in which this specialty is now practised. There is also a chapter on evaluating palliative care services, including a more detailed review of quality-of-life issues, audit and the evidence for effectiveness of various services. Finally, several ethical issues are discussed, including end-of-life treatment decisions and euthanasia. Throughout the book, cultural diversity is addressed, as well as the potentially difficult overlap between anti-cancer treatments and palliative care.

Acknowledgement

We gratefully acknowledge the contributions of Dr Nigel Sykes, FRCGP and Dr Mary Baines, FRCP who are the authors of Chapter 4 (*Gastro-intestinal Symptoms in Oncology*).

London, September 1997   Robert Dunlop

1 – Evolution of Palliative Care

Introduction

The twentieth century has seen a dramatic increase in medical advances. Cures are now possible for many illnesses, life expectancy has been extended for other chronic diseases, and, even when treatment is not possible, the pathophysiology of the condition is likely to be understood. These advances in medical science have bought new life and hope for many patients.

The management of cancer illustrates how dramatic the changes have been. Technological advances have improved the accuracy of staging and diagnosis. Improvements have also occurred in surgical techniques, radiotherapy treatments, and chemotherapy regimens. More cancers are now curable, and research is continuing to produce even more options. Supportive measures, such as antiemetic therapy, platelet transfusions and stimulants of white cell production, can reduce the morbidity from treatment. Yet, despite all these advances, most cancer patients still die of their disease and cancer remains a leading cause of death.

This book is about palliative care, a newly emerged speciality in the field of cancer medicine. Palliative care is the care of patients who have progressive incurable disease and the care of their families. This speciality has also had a major impact on the practice of medicine generally. No longer should dying patients have to summon the courage to interrupt a nurse, only to find that pain-killers are not available, nor should they have to silently suffer their dark and terrible fears. Relatives can find support for their anguish, the strength to cope, and the capacity to recover after the patient dies. Even in the face of incurable disease, when there is nothing more that can be done with anti-cancer treatment, patients can still find meaning and purpose to their living. When health-care professionals become aware of what palliative care can do, they become more interested in the challenges these patients present. Their clinical relationships with patients and families become more satisfying, more complete. The principles of palliative care then carry over to the care of patients who have curable diseases as well.

In this chapter, a brief historical review of the care of dying patients is presented. This will place the origins of the modern hospice movement into context. The principles of palliative are also outlined.

The Historical Background to Palliative Care

It is often said that the dying became neglected with the introduction of high-technology medicine, as epitomised by the use of artificial ventilation to keep alive patients with severe irreversible brain damage. The use of aggressive chemotherapy regimens or bone marrow transplantation, when there is virtually no hope of cure, are also held out by some as examples of science overwhelming the 'art' of medicine. A careful review of the history of hospital care shows that the problems of dying patients go back over centuries, long before medicine even became a recognised discipline.

The earliest hospitals in England were founded by religious orders. The oldest medieval hospital still on its original site is St Bartholomew's Hospital, founded in 1123 by the monk Rahere. He established the hospital in association with a priory which helped to manage the finances and operation of the hospital. The original hospital comprised a large hall built near the chapel. The hall was used to provide rest and shelter for the sick poor of London. The master of the priory visited the patients daily. Volunteers were used to help care for the patients. The public also gave charitable donations of money and food.

Although medications and treatments were very rudimentary, it was not long before St Bartholomew's Hospital became known as a place where people could be cured. Within two decades of opening, the earliest documents reported patients who received miraculous healing, such as the woman whose swollen tongue resolved when Rahere placed a relic of the Cross upon it, the man who had a headache relieved, and a cripple who was able to walk again. This leads to patients travelling from all over England in search of treatment.

By the sixteenth century, the emphasis on cure was so well established that it was included in the equivalent of a 'mission statement' – the hospital was

> '(f)or the ayde and comforte of the poore, sykke, blynde, aged, and impotent persones beying not hable to helpe themselffs nor havying any place certeyn whereyn they may be lodged, cherysshed or refresshed, tyll they be cured and holpen of theyre dyseases and syknesse.'   (Moore, 1918)

One of the job descriptions written at the same time as the Mission Statement illustrates how the attitudes to cure were jeopardising the care of dying patients. At this time, when surgery existed as a separate speciality but with a very limited repertoire, a key role of the surgeons was 'to see if the patient were curable or not, so that none should be admitted who were incurable, none rejected who were curable' (Moore, 1918).

The birth of the Age of Reason saw the influence of Gallen's dogmas on medical thinking give way to the systematic analysis of anatomy and physiology, the categorisation of diseases, and the discovery of new therapies. Cartesian philosophy, which emphasised the dualistic nature of the body and the mind, provided the basis for scientific thinking to break from the influence of theology and the Church. These new directions resulted in rapid advances in the practice of medicine, but at a cost to care. The spiritual view of patients was replaced by the medical model of illness with its focus on the physical. This provided doctors with an intellectual barrier that dulled awareness of the broader aspects of suffering. The rational approach to medicine only added to the already established marginalisation of the dying. This suggests that the factors which lead to terminally ill patients being shunned are the deep-seated, primitive fears associated with death and dying, the overwhelming sense of helplessness and distress that arises from watching someone who is suffering, rather than the fact that medicine became a science.

The Modern Hospice Movement

Hospices originated in the Middle Ages. Like hospitals, they were also built by religious orders but were used to provide places of rest and refuge for pilgrims. In keeping with the derivation of the word 'hospice' from the Latin word for hospitality, hospices provided entertainment and food, as well as shelter.

It was not until the middle of the nineteenth century that Madame Jeanne Garnier opened the first hospice for the dying in France. Shortly afterwards, hospices were built in Eire and England. The hospice in County Cork was established to improve the care of patients dying of cancer, following a distressing personal experience by the founder. However, many of the hospices were founded to cope with the increasing numbers of the poor dying from tuberculosis who were not being admitted to hospitals.

The early hospices remained isolated from main-stream medicine. Some important innovations in care were developed, such as the regular administration of oral morphine for cancer pain in St Luke's Home for the Dying Poor, London. However, these developments were not transferred back into hospital practice. Few hospice practitioners emulated Dr Howard Barrett, founder of St Luke's, who attempted to raise the profile of terminal care. The public were often unaware of the existence of hospices, except when they lived nearby. For those people living in the vicinity, hospices were often associated with powerful negative connotations. For example, children would be encouraged to run past the entrance lest the nuns reach out and grab them, pulling them into the place of death, the place of no hope. These deep-seated fears still exist in the minds of some people today.

By the 1960s, the physical environment within many hospices had become unsatisfactory. The nurses were dedicated but their care was compromised by overcrowded conditions, poor facilities and financial constraints. In one hospice, the lift was too small for a bed. Once a patient had become bedbound, he or she could not be transferred off the ward until after death.

Hospice care took on a new dimension when Dame Cicely Saunders opened St Christopher's Hospice in 1967. She had become aware of the needs of dying patients while working as a nurse and then an almoner. Her determination to relieve the distress of these patients led her to become a doctor. Dr Saunders then came across the use of regular morphine at St Luke's. She studied this practice carefully, showing that opioids could relieve pain when given orally and that tolerance was not a problem when the dose was individually titrated. However,

Dr Saunders realised that the effective use of morphine was not of itself enough to improve the overall care of the terminally ill. The caring art of medicine needed to be restored along with the sensitive application of the scientific method. Furthermore, the new-found knowledge and expertise needed to be widely disseminated.

The in-patient unit of St Christopher's Hospice was purpose built for research and teaching as well as clinical care. It was this combination of functions which marked the beginning of the modern hospice movement. As staff learned more about the needs of patients and families, the hospice rapidly expanded to provide home care and bereavement follow-up services. The work became more widely known and other people adapted the example of St Christopher's Hospice into many different settings, including acute hospitals and nursing homes. Some of the developments included palliative-care units providing hospice beds within hospitals, home-care advisory teams, and support teams in hospitals. Many of these innovations were developed in the voluntary sector, without government funding. There are now hundreds of palliative-care services throughout the United Kingdom. The hospice movement has been adjusted to suit different cultures and has spread world wide, testifying to the universal need that exists. There can be no doubt about the enormous impact of palliative care.

The term 'Palliative Care' was coined soon after the hospice movement began. It was used to overcome some of the limitations of the word 'hospice' when describing the broad application of the knowledge and skills developed at St Christopher's. 'Hospice' was often associated with the image of a building rather than with a concept of care. This reflected the prior existence in many countries of hospice units which had been founded by religious orders. The focus of these units had been on the care of dying patients, which led to a narrow interpretation of when 'hospice' care was appropriate. It had also fostered the myths and misconceptions in the minds of lay-people described earlier. Although these misinterpretations were based largely on ignorance, they reflected people's deep-rooted fear of death and constituted a significant barrier to the dissemination of the modern hospice movement.

'Palliative' is derived from 'pallium' which is the Latin word for a cloak. The image of a cloak as a superficial covering hiding what is underneath is an excellent depiction of hospice care. If a patient has an irremediable and progressive disease, treatments aimed at cure will be inappropriate. Such treatments may make the patient feel worse. The aim of care then has to be redirected at controlling the effects of the illness on the patient and the family. This concept has been included in the World Health Organization's definition of palliative care:

> 'The active total care of patients whose disease is not responsive to curative treatment. Control of pain, of other symptoms, and of psychological, social, and spiritual problems is paramount. The goal of palliative care is achievement of the best quality of life for patients and their families. Many aspects of palliative care are also applicable earlier in the course of the illness in conjunction with anticancer treatment.' (World Health Organization, 1990)

The term 'palliative' is used in the oncology setting as well. However, it has a different meaning which has caused some confusion and misunderstanding between oncology and hospice services. Cancer specialists use 'palliative' to describe anti-cancer treatments such as radiotherapy, chemotherapy and surgery which are being used for patients with incurable cancer. The aim of 'palliative' treatment is to reduce the cancer as much as possible even though cure is not possible. If the tumour bulk is reduced by the treatment, improvement in symptoms may occur until the cancer regrows. However, 'palliative' anti-cancer therapies do not always control symptoms, in which case additional symptom control measures will be necessary. The cancer may be resistant to the treatment. Another example would be if a tumour produces pain by the collapsing of a vertebra. Even if the cancer is destroyed locally, the structural integrity of the vertebra may be so disrupted that pain continues despite successful 'palliation' of the cancer. For the purposes of clarity, whenever the word 'palliative' immediately precedes one of the disease-modifying treatments, as in 'palliative radiotherapy' or 'palliative chemotherapy', the more restricted meaning described in this paragraph will apply. However, even in these instances, the broader aims of palliative care should always be borne in mind. It is the wider definition that is intended whenever the word 'palliative' is otherwise used.

The oncological meaning of 'palliative' is based on a biomedical model of cancer. This model neglects the wider psychological, social and spiritual perspectives which, in turn, causes problems in patient care. These problems were recently highlighted in a paper published by Cleeland et al. (1994). They undertook a detailed study of pain management in patients receiving anti-cancer treatments at centres within the Eastern Cooperative Oncology Group (ECOG). Many patients were experiencing severe pain, despite the fact that oncologists were more aware than other doctors of the treatments for cancer pain. This study also showed that non-medical factors were obviously influencing treatment decisions. Young women, elderly patients and patients from ethnic minorities were even less likely to have adequate pain control.

Palliative care offers an enhancement to the biomedical model, not in opposition, but as a further resource for those seeking to improve existing practice. Hospices use skilled awareness and treatment of a patient's symptoms and feelings to achieve the maximum potential in personal capacity and in social relationships. They have defined the standard of care that is achievable, by specialising in the care of patients with intractable physical, emotional or social problems. However, the majority of patients will continue to die at home or in acute hospitals. Effective palliative care, guided by the principles set out in Table 1.1, should be available to all patients no matter what the setting.

Table 1.1 Principles of palliative care

1. Patient and family are the 'unit of care'
2. Attention to physical, psychological, social and spiritual needs
3. Multi-professional teamwork
4. Evaluation of care
5. 24-hour, 7-days a week availability
6. Support during bereavement
7. Education and teaching
8. Therapeutic physical environment
9. Care of patients with non-malignant conditions
10. Supportive administration
11. Preparedness for the cost of care

The Patient and the Family Comprise the 'Unit of Care'

Cancer, indeed any illness, does not just affect the patient. The impact will encompass family, friends and significant others. Their reactions will, in turn, feed back to the patient. Therefore problems caused by cancer can only be wholly managed if the patient and family are actively involved. Health-care professionals must deliberately become refocused to achieve this. For example, medical consultations usually take place in a doctor's surgery, out-patient clinic or an acute ward without the family being present. Patients frequently under-report their symptoms because they do not want to 'upset' or 'bother' the doctor. The observations of the family should be actively sought, although their views should not be allowed to override those of the patient. Time must also be made available, usually on several occasions, for families to ask questions and to express fears and concerns. Patient confidentiality must be respected but most patients appreciate having family members present when important clinical issues are discussed. Even if the patient refuses to allow information to be shared, it is possible to allow the relatives to voice their worries without compromising patient confidentiality.

Attention to Physical, Psychological, Social and Spiritual Needs

The lives of patients and families are affected in many ways by cancer. Physical symptoms, psycho-social needs and spiritual concerns are present throughout the illness. The nature and intensity of these problems will vary; there will be the shock of the initial diagnosis, the impact of coping with treatment, then the adaptation to a period of remission followed by the disappointment when a recurrence is diagnosed and then the increasing difficulties of the final phase of the illness. This book will focus on the latter stage which may last days, weeks or, occasionally, months.

The Needs of Patients – Symptom Control

Several studies have documented the symptoms of patients with advanced malignancies. Most patients have several distressing symptoms. Pain, anorexia, weakness, constipation and breathlessness are experienced by most patients. Other symptoms include nausea, vomiting, sore mouth, cough, haemoptysis and dysphagia. The frequency and severity of these symptoms increases throughout the terminal phase. Insomnia is a common problem for patients in hospital wards. Drowsiness, agitation and confusion become more frequent in the final days of life.

Unfortunately, too many patients still suffer from unrelieved symptoms. There are several reasons why symptoms are poorly managed. Patients and families frequently accept symptoms as inevitable and do not complain. Professionals fail to specifically ask about symptoms, especially those that are not readily obvious, such as nausea, pain and constipation. Even when symptoms are recognised, treatments are often inappropriate, for example, the all too common prescribing of inadequate and infrequent doses of analgesics and laxatives.

The treatment of physical symptoms is reviewed in Chapters 2, 3, 4 and 5. Chapter 9 deals with the ethical basis for making treatment decisions and with ethical dilemmas commonly encountered in terminal care.

Psychological and Spiritual Needs

Cancer patients experience a wide range of disturbing emotions. Hinton (1963) found that at least 50% of terminally ill patients in hospital described themselves as feeling depressed, especially if they were experiencing several distressing symptoms or were aware that they were dying. He found that at least 75% of patients were aware of their impending death, even if they had not been given a diagnosis. The distinction between appropriate sadness and clinical depression can be very difficult when patients have physical symptoms from advanced cancer.

Anxiety is another common emotion, particularly when patients are not told of their diagnosis. Most patients want to be told the nature of their disease and want to know about their prognosis (Mount and Scott, 1983). However, there is a small group of patients for whom disclosure will cause distress. Breaking bad news requires skill and tact.

Anxiety is also associated with some symptoms, particularly breathlessness. Patients who have dependants will often be very anxious. Other sources of patient stress include the lengthy periods waiting for results of investigations or treatments for cancer and the complex technologies used for treatment and diagnosis.

Other strong emotions, such as guilt and anger, are encountered less often. The latter can be very difficult to deal with, especially if there were delays in making the diagnosis. The recognition and management of psychological problems is dealt with in a forthcoming book in this series on psychological care. This book will also cover the breaking of bad news.

A terminal illness will raise many profound existential issues for patients. Questions such as 'Why me?' and 'What have I done to deserve this?' are common and represent a search for some sense of meaning. Patients with a strong religious faith may question the existence of God; other patients may feel guilty and fearful because they have drifted away from a religious upbringing. For some, there is a sense of despair and hopelessness without any religious connotations. The recognition and management of spiritual pain is considered in Chapter 8.

The Needs of Relatives – Physical Symptoms

When cancer patients become weaker, relatives perform most of the personal cares. Patients eventually require assistance with dressing, eating, washing and getting out of bed. The physical effort, coupled with the stress of coping, exact a heavy toll on carers. Fatigue is the most common symptom experienced by them. As many as 20% of relatives will develop a physical illness.

Relatives continue to experience physical symptoms during the bereavement period. Sleeplessness, palpitations, fatigue, chest discomfort, loss of appetite and weight loss are some of the problems which are frequently reported to general practitioners in the months after the patient dies. Some relatives complain of the symptoms experienced by the patient.

Psychological Needs

Carers experience many distressing emotions. They can feel depressed and anxious at the prospect of losing the patient. These feelings are heightened when patients want to talk about dying. Relatives find themselves changing the subject or trying to be optimistic, only to feel more depressed because of the breakdown in a trusting relationship. Anger is not common, but when it is does occur, it is often deflected away from the immediate situation on to perceived delays in diagnosis or social problems, such as difficulties in transport, or on to the health-care professionals. In addition to their own distress, carers often have to cope with the negative feelings and frustrations of the patients as well. Patients often hide their feelings from visitors then vent them on the relatives.

Fear is another important symptom experienced by many relatives. They are frightened by patients' distressing symptoms. Relatives are also afraid that patients will fall or die at home. These fears are exacerbated when there is a perceived lack of general practitioner support. The combination of fear, helplessness and sense of responsibility often thwart efforts to care for patients at home. If hospitalisation is required, relatives feel guilty because they have let the patient down.

Lack of information makes these emotions worse. This is a major problem when patients are in hospital, which is where the diagnosis of cancer is usually made. Relatives receive conflicting statements about the patient's condition and prognosis (Hockley et al., 1988). Relatives may be desperate for more information but they are usually too afraid to disrupt the routine of the doctors and nurses. Poor communication also results from the frequent changes in junior medical staff.

The distress caused by relatives' unmet needs is reflected in the degree to which they will criticise the hospital as being uncaring. Wilkes (1984) found that one-fifth of relatives were critical when followed up several months after the patients had died. The memories often remain very vivid and painful for years. Relatives find it difficult to make a complaint, but a high proportion of written grievances received by hospitals relate to the care of dying patients.

Social Needs

The structure and integrity of the patient and family unit are threatened by the effects of cancer. Loss of earning power will have important financial consequences for younger patients. Older patients are often unaware of the benefits to which they may be entitled. Relationships will be disrupted by redistribution of roles, and by changes in the patient's sexuality. Social isolation is common.

Patients may be too weak to get out and carers too frightened to leave the patients at home. Friends and relations are often uncertain about how to relate to the patient, further compounding the social isolation. The needs of the patients' children are often overlooked. Their grief may find expression in the classroom or in disruptive behaviour at home. Health-care professionals must make a determined effort to discover these broader non-medical issues.

Multi-Disciplinary Teamwork

The variety and complexity of problems described above cannot be managed by any single health-care professional. Quite apart from the levels of skill and knowledge that are required, palliative care is very time-intensive. Doctors, nurses, social workers, physiotherapists, occupational therapists, clergy and pharmacists all have a role to play. Hospices make extensive use of volunteers as well. In the hospital and the hospice setting, the expertise of oncologists, radio-therapists, anaesthetists and psychiatrists may be required. In the community setting, Jones (1993) demonstrated that a team approach comprising general practitioner, district nurse and specialist (Macmillan) nurse provided better symptom control for terminally ill cancer patients than general practitioners operating alone.

Effective team working depends upon having goals which are understood and shared by all of the members, effective communication between disciplines and a clear understanding of roles. Palliative care has encouraged multi-skilling across disciplines. For example, nurses are able to assess pain, make limited diagnoses such as pain arising from pressure areas, and can review pain therapy. They can also provide support and counselling, helping the patient and family to understand and cope with the pain and its treatment. Not surprisingly, multi-skilling may lead to role conflict. Experienced and confident leadership is needed to ensure maximum team effectiveness. A review of team working is contained in Chapter 10.

Evaluation of Care

St Christopher's Hospice was founded on the methodical recording and analysis of clinical practice. Early research into the use of oral opioids proved to be the springboard for launching palliative care. Other health-care professionals recognised and responded to legitimate academic achievement. The emphasis on research has continued, yielding new insights and treatments as well as refining existing strategies.

The prospect of research raises many concerns: the need for rigorous protocols, ethical committee approval, research assistants and funding. Only a few palliative-care services will be able to conduct research. However, even the smallest service should evaluate what it is doing. Clinical audit is becoming widely practised as government funding agencies demand more evidence of improvements in all sectors of health care. Audit should not be seen as a means of appeasing the funding authorities but rather as an opportunity for identifying deficiencies in care, effecting improvements in service and providing evidence of good practice which can be used to give positive feedback to staff.

Chapter 12 identifies some of the problems which hamper research into palliative care and reviews the studies which have evaluated palliative care. Clinical audit is also discussed.

Twenty-Four Hour, Seven Days a Week Availability

Terminally ill patients and their families can experience problems at any time of the day or night. The night time is particularly difficult because it heightens feelings of loneliness and fear. Support must be constantly available from health-care professionals who know the patient and family. This is always possible in the hospice in-patient setting but patients spend most of their last months at home. In the community, home-care teams must be developed and fully integrated with the existing community services. The patient's own doctor usually remains in charge, using the hospice team as a resource. Plans for after-hours support must be clearly established and communicated to the patient and family. If a patient is to be discharged home or requires admission to a general hospital or hospice bed, every effort must be made to ensure smooth continuity of care.

Support During Bereavement

The effect of an illness like cancer does not end when the patient dies. The family must go through a period of mourning and then gradual recovery. Not every relative needs support – other members of the family, neighbours, spiritual advisors and family doctors – can often provide all the help that is necessary. Palliative-care services must be able to identify those with special needs, then provide the support or refer the relative to an existing bereavement service for counselling. Many hospices use trained volunteers to provide skilled unhurried listening. This can reduce the considerable morbidity experienced by bereaved people. Grief and bereavement are considered in Chapter 7.

Education and Teaching

Palliative-care teams need to exploit every opportunity for teaching about terminal care. Teaching can occur in many ways. Written papers, lectures, seminars and other formal methods are commonly used by larger hospices with teaching programmes. Practical experience can be gained by working in these units. Most hospices also provide an informal telephone consultation service. Advisory palliative-care teams working in hospitals or the community rely on the informal opportunities that arise while working alongside other health-care professionals. Not only do the team members provide a practical example of how to deliver palliative care, but they can also base teaching on individual patient problems which are current and fresh in the minds of their colleagues. Community teams make frequent contact with nurses and doctors from the primary-health-care teams to pick up openings for teaching and support. Hospital-based services can use existing forums for teaching, such as grand rounds. Teaching hospitals provide an ideal chance for reaching students in all disciplines while they are still impressionable.

The content of a teaching session must be geared to the recipients. Students often need advice on talking to cancer patients and handling their emotional reactions. The principles of symptom control can also be taught early on, emphasising the importance of seeking advice as well increasing awareness of the therapeutic options. More senior staff need practical teaching on breaking bad news and supporting patients and families.

Therapeutic Physical Environment

Advisory palliative-care teams working in hospitals or in the community usually do not have any beds of their own. Hospice in-patient units will have beds in a purpose-built or a renovated building. Palliative-care units have beds which are dedicated to palliative care in a general hospital. Whatever the physical location, the architecture must be used imaginatively, combining privacy for patients, families and staff with efficient and easy clinical and domestic care. Interior decorations must be soothing and home-like; the external environment should be aesthetically pleasing and engender tranquillity. With vision, perseverance and creativity, these effects can even be achieved in hospitals.

Care of Patients with Non-Malignant Diseases

Only a quarter of all deaths are due to cancer. There are many other disadvantaged patient groups who need the same focus and attention. Patients with non-malignant diseases are just as likely to have symptoms but are much less likely than cancer patients to have these symptoms controlled. Hospital-based services are more liable to be referred patients with stroke, heart disease, respiratory conditions and uncommon illnesses. Some hospices treat long-term progressive illnesses, such as motor neurone disease. There is increasing awareness of the growing population of frail elderly and the need to provide support and advice when these patients are cared for in nursing homes. This book does not deal with palliative care for patients with non-malignant conditions but many of the general principles can be carried over.

Supportive Administration

Palliative-care services are managed in several ways. Independent hospices often have personnel with dedicated administrative roles This reflects the size of these units and their need to maintain fundraising and public relations functions for survival. In this situation, an efficient and approachable administration is necessary to provide security for patients, families and staff. Community-based palliative-care services may be linked managerially to the local hospice, but many are managed in the non-voluntary sector. Hospital-based advisory teams also usually operate in the non-voluntary sector. Lines of management are usually drawn to existing service directorates such as oncology, medicine or community support services. The managers should have an understanding of, and dedication to, palliative care.

Preparedness for the Cost of Care

An outstanding characteristic of the staff in hospices past and present has been their devotion to care. Palliative care is demanding. Anyone who is seriously interested in this work must be prepared for the cost of commitment. It is not easy to support patients and families as they struggle to find meaning in the face of a devastating illness. They may come to some understanding but it is often incomplete and unsatisfying. Staff are confronted with strong emotions and their own mortality is brought sharply to the fore. Yet, for all these challenges and difficulties, palliative care can be immensely rewarding. This book can only provide a glimpse into the challenges and rewards, but there can be no question that palliative care has fundamentally changed the practice of medicine. For anyone who is interested in this field, be encouraged to pursue this interest – your dealings with patients, families and colleagues will never be the same again.

2 – Management of Pain

Introduction

Cancer and pain are synonymous in the minds of the public. The thought of an agonising death is still one of the most feared outcomes of cancer. Pain is a common symptom but it is not inevitable. One-third of patients present with pain at diagnosis but the incidence increases to more than two-thirds of patients who are terminally ill. Patients who are dying tolerate all symptoms poorly, especially pain. Pain must be recognised, assessed and treated promptly. There is growing evidence drawn from large clinical series and from many different countries which clearly shows that cancer pain can be relieve (e.g. Schug et al., 1990). Pharmacological measures form the mainstay of treatment but this chapter will also review the non-pharmacological strategies which are available.

Pain is not a single entity. There are many different types of pain and most patients will experience more than one pain. Each pain will have physical, as well as emotional and social consequences, that must be carefully assessed while management is being planned. Psycho-social and spiritual influences have a powerful effect on pain perception and upon the treatments which the patient and family will accept and respond to. Some patients will have pain that is not caused by the cancer. Non-malignant causes for pain in cancer patients include treatments such as surgery, diseases such as shingles, and the range of painful conditions which affect people generally, such as osteoarthritis. These issues emphasise the need for a detailed clinical evaluation of each pain. The process for evaluating pain will be described in detail in this chapter. It can also be applied to the assessment of the other symptoms discussed in this book.

The careful assessment of a pain problem will guide further treatment. Most pains can be classified according to the tissues involved: superficial somatic, deep somatic, visceral or neuropathic. These classifications are discussed in more detail, along with the most appropriate treatments.

This chapter highlights some of the general principles for managing cancer pain which also apply when treating other symptoms. Because the patient and the family must be thought of as the unit of care, the care-givers also need support and encouragement. A collaborative multi-disciplinary approach by health-care professionals is needed to achieve this. Regular and continued follow-up is needed to ensure that the treatment is working, to alert the team to new symptoms, and to maintain support. If pain is not controlled, early involvement of specialist services should be considered.

Multi-Disciplinary Team Working

The multi-faceted nature of a patient's pain experience, coupled with the distressing impact on the family, requires a team approach from doctors, nurses and other disciplines. No single health-care professional can have the experience, expertise, and especially the time, needed to address all of the problems. Effective multi-disciplinary working is difficult but it begins by recognising that the needs of the patient and family are central. Their needs and perceptions must guide the efforts of the team. There has to be a high degree of communication between disciplines which must be constantly worked on.

Palliative care promotes expanded roles for the various disciplines. Doctors have traditionally been responsible for diagnosing and treating pain. With training and support, nurses and physiotherapists can assess pain in the community and in hospitals. Skilled non-medical practitioners can even make limited diagnoses, for example, by raising the suspicion of bone metastases or identifying pain arising from pressure areas. This does not replace the role of the doctor as diagnostician but supplements it, making the doctor's interaction with the patient more effective and efficient. Nurses can review pain therapy, being able to visit more frequently and spend more time with the patients and families. They can advise on changes in pain therapy and provide valuable feedback to the doctor. Social workers and spiritual advisors have important adjunctive roles in assessing the patient and family dynamics, along with providing support and counselling.

Assessment of Pain

A careful pain assessment is needed every time a patient presents with a new pain (see Table 2.1). Because cancer patients frequently have more than one pain, each pain should be appraised separately. Pain is a subjective experience. This means that the patient's perspective is essential. Patients often under-report their pain to doctors. There are many reasons for this. Sometimes the patient accepts that pain is inevitable, sometimes acknowledging the pain means acknowledging that the cancer is active and the patient prefers denial. However, the most common reason is that patients have difficulty telling health-care professionals because they do not want to 'upset' or 'bother' them. This is especially likely in a busy clinic or family practice. It is important for health-care professionals not to give the impression of being rushed. If it is not possible to allow sufficient time in the clinical interview, then make another appointment, or visit the person at home. Doctors should enlist the help of other professionals such as a nurse who can make domiciliary calls. When appropriate, confirm what the patient has said with the observations of the family.

The first step is to take a thorough history of the pain. The patient should be asked to describe where the pain is located and where it radiates to. The onset of the pain should be established, along with some understanding of the temporal pattern: is the pain constant, fluctuating, paroxysmal or intermittent? If the pain is not constant, find out what the frequency and periodicity is. The pain intensity can be gauged by asking whether the patient would describe the pain as mild, moderate or severe. Open-ended questions should be used to encourage the patient to give a qualitative description. If the pain is described as 'sharp', check whether the meaning is the qualitative *like a pin-prick* or whether it is the quantitative *severe*. Some people have trouble describing the qualitative nature of pain. Offering them a list of words such as dull, aching, burning, stabbing and throbbing can be helpful. Relieving and aggravating factors should be identified, including the responses to previous treatments. Sleep disturbance caused by pain is a very serious symptom.

Table 2.1   Assessment of pain in cancer patients

1. Thorough pain history:
   - site
   - radiation
   - onset and temporal pattern
   - qualitative description
   - relieving and aggravating factors
   - sleep disturbance
2. Record pain history and assessment on pain chart
3. Past and current history of cancer
4. Physical examination:
   - pain behaviour (signs of acute pain often absent)
   - site/s of pain
   - other features, e.g. organomegaly
   - spinal cord function when indicated
5. Appropriate investigations

Some attempt should be made to establish the past and current history of cancer. A pain chart can be used to record the pain history and assessment. For audit purposes, a simple numerical analogue scale may be sufficient, with the patient rating the pain from zero meaning 'no pain' through to 10 correlating with the 'worst possible pain'. Visual analogue scales (VASs) have been widely used, but are difficult for older patients to understand. The VAS consists of a line measuring exactly 10 cm with the anchors 'no pain' and 'worst possible pain' at either end. The patient draws a mark on the line corresponding to the pain intensity which can then be translated into a distance measurement. Most pain charts have an outline of the front and back of a body upon which the patient can draw the location of the pain. A new pain may correspond with the site of known metastases. For example, a past bone scan may be indicated by increased uptake in the spine which was not previously painful. The type of cancer will also predict where metastases are likely to occur, thereby heightening clinical suspicion. Past treatments may cause pain, for example, scar pain in a post-mastectomy patient.

Causes other than cancer must be borne in mind. Just because a patient has a past history of cancer, or even has evidence of active disease, does not mean that every symptom is due to the cancer. Shingles may cause pain in cancer patients. Cancer is more common in older patients, so are other conditions such as osteoarthritis, ischaemic heart disease and chronic pulmonary disease, which may all cause symptoms that mimic cancer.

The next step in the assessment process is a physical examination. This step becomes more important if the patient is too ill or too confused to give a history. Non-medical staff can also gain a lot of information from examining a patient. The general appearance and behaviour of the patient may give valuable clues, for example, wincing and groaning when turned or touched. The site or sites of pain should be checked for tenderness, inflammation and altered sensation. Gently stroking or touching the skin may reveal an area of numbness or heightened sensitivity in keeping with nerve damage. Another sign of nerve damage is allodynia, when light touch produces pain. Deeper palpation may reveal lymph node enlargement, organomegaly, or the presence of a mass. If the patient gives a story of back or neck pain, spinal cord function must be checked to exclude cord compression. This will produce motor weakness, a sensory level, incompetence of rectal sphincter and bladder distension from retention. The behavioural signs of acute pain such as pallor, sweating and rapid breathing, are rarely present in patients with chronic cancer pain. This has often led to the erroneous judgement that a patient cannot be experiencing the severe pain he or she is describing because the signs of acute pain are not visible.

A psycho-social assessment is also important. This requires time, often on several occasions, for the patient and family to talk about the meaning and impact of the pain. For example, some people view pain as a sign that the patient is about to die, or as a punishment for past wrong-doing. Cultural and religious belief systems are powerful determinants of patient and family perceptions; it is often necessary to draw on the expertise of others to help interpret these effects. Past experiences, especially of relatives or friends who have died of cancer, should be enquired into. Preferences for, and concerns about, treatment are important. The use of morphine, for example, often reinforces the idea that the patient is imminently dying. If this fear is not addressed, the morphine will be withheld and treatment will be ineffective. Uncontrolled cancer pain is often associated with mood changes such as depression, anger, fear and guilt, all of which decrease the pain threshold. Any psycho-social assessment must enquire into the effects of the pain on the family. They will often vividly describe the sense of helplessness at having to watch someone suffering, the perceived lack of social support and the impact of changing financial and inter-personal circumstances. Always check that the patient and family have sufficient information about the pain.

There are several groups of patients who deserve extra attention and time because they are less likely to get adequate pain relief. Ethnic minorities and people with existing drug dependency problems are particularly at risk. Women, especially young women, also had more pain in the previously mentioned study by Cleeland et al. (1994). The elderly are at risk for many reasons: they are often considered incapable of experiencing severe pain, and they are more likely to be confused and unable to give a pain history. Behavioural signs of pain may be more important in this group (Ferrell, 1991).

Diagnostic tests may help to find the cause of a particular pain but these must be tailored to the physical condition of the patient. Patients who are imminently dying should not be subjected to unnecessary and distressing tests – a clinical diagnosis will be quite adequate. If the patient is well enough, the appropriate use of x-rays, bone scans, ultrasound scans, CT or MRI scans will often help confirm the cause of a pain. It is very important not to withhold pain treatment until a diagnosis is confirmed. Too often patients are left to suffer pain while undergoing tests and, worse still, while awaiting results. It is always possible to start analgesic therapy after the initial clinical assessment.

General Principles of Treatment

Before discussing specific therapies, it is important to emphasise some general principles. The first important principle in the treatment of any symptom has already been covered: a careful clinical review to establish a working diagnosis. This enables the most appropriate treatments to be selected and avoids wasting time with drugs which are unlikely to work. Table 2.3 illustrates the other principles which are covered in this section.

Table 2.3   General principles of cancer pain

1. Careful clinical review
2. Consider anti-cancer treatments
3. Give regular medication for chronic symptoms
4. Treatments should be individually tailored
5. Choose convenient preparations, preferably by oral route
6. Use a logical, step-wise approach
7. Write down and explain the treatment plan
8. Regular follow-up

Whenever possible, treatment directed at controlling the cancer should be considered for symptoms that are caused by cancer. Surgery may have an immediate effect on the symptoms but radiotherapy, chemotherapy and hormone manipulation usually take several days to weeks before symptom control is apparent from regression of the cancer. Therefore, if anti-cancer treatments are an option, patients should be given other symptom-control measures, such as adequate doses of analgesics, while a treatment response is awaited. Many patients, particularly those with advanced disease, will have had maximum possible anti-cancer therapy or will be too ill. For these patients, pharmacological therapy is the mainstay of pain management.

Most symptoms from cancer are constant and unremitting. Treatments must be given regularly, first to relieve, and then to prevent, the symptom from recurring. There is no place for the use of 'as required' medications for chronic symptoms. Numerous studies have shown that if a patient needs to ask for treatment when the symptom recurs, there will be delays in receiving it. This results in the symptom getting worse and an escalation in drug dosage. There are three key goals for the treatment of pain: relief of pain at night, then at rest, and, most difficult of all, freedom of pain on movement. These goals must be set in the context of trying to maintain the maximum possible quality of life and independence for the patient.

Treatment must be individually tailored for each patient. Patients with advanced cancer are generally less tolerant of side-effects. Elderly patients need lower doses of most drugs because of altered distribution, greater sensitive to side-effects and reduced drug clearance. Longer dosing intervals may need to be considered if drug accumulation occurs. If reduced drug clearance is anticipated, it is often appropriate to delay a decision on a dose increase to allow for time for the drug to reach steady state.

Terminally ill patients have multiple symptoms requiring many different medications. Wherever possible, once- or twice-daily preparations should be used. This reduces the number of tablets and maximises the preventative effect. If a range of choices is available in any drug category, e.g. NSAIDs, choose preparations that are easy to swallow. Sick patients have difficulty swallowing large uncoated tablets. When a range of drug categories is available for one symptom, the choice should take into account other symptoms. For example, a patient with neuropathic pain and anxiety could be started on the benzodi-azepene clonazepam, whereas a patient with neuropathic pain and loss of appetite could be started on steroids.

The treatment for most symptoms can be based on a logical stepwise approach. The current recommendations from the World Health Organization (1990) offer the best example of this. Several multinational trials have validated the so-called 'step ladder' method of treating cancer pain (see Table 3.3). This method was designed to provide maximum pain control in countries with limited health-care resources. Patients are started on the treatment ladder at the level commensurate with the pain severity, progressing to the next step if the pain is not controlled after an adequate trial period. The first step on the ladder is the use of simple analgesics such as paracetamol combined with a non-steroidal anti-inflammatory drug (NSAID). If the pain is not controlled, the next step is to add a weak opioid such as codeine. The final step is to substitute a strong opioid, usually morphine, for the weak opioid. At all steps, adjuvant treatments such as radiotherapy for bone pain or hyoscine for colic, should be considered.

Table 3.4   WHO analgesic step-ladder

1. Simple analgesics:
   (a) paracetamol (acetaminophen)
   (b) NSAID
2. Weak opioid – e.g. codeine
3. Strong opioid – e.g. morphine

N.B.: Adjuvants used for specific pain problems

The treatment plan should always be written down for the patient and family. The plan should include the names of any medications, the indications for each drug, dosages and timing, what should be done if symptoms recur or escalate, and strategies for avoiding side-effects, for example, the regular use of laxatives with opioids. In the home setting, contact telephone numbers should be available for trained health-care professionals who are familiar with the situation.

The final principle of symptom management is regular follow-up. As cancer progresses, an increase in number and severity of symptoms is likely. This reinforces the need for frequent reviews to make sure that treatments have been effective, to elicit any side-effects, to review the treatment plan, to provide encouragement and to detect new symptoms. Contact should be made daily or more often until new symptoms are controlled, especially if they are severe. Visits or telephone contacts can then be made less often. If a symptom, such as pain, recurs, the situation should be reassessed. A new pain will require evaluation and possibly different treatment, an existing pain which has become worse may just require an increase in the usual medication. Follow-up contacts should allow time for ongoing support for patients and families, a vital part of any treatment plan. This includes updating information about the illness and the symptoms, instruction and support in providing physical care, praise and encouragement, assistance with practical and financial needs, and the opportunity to share feelings and concerns.

Common Pain Problems in Cancer Patients

There are many different ways of classifying pain. One of the most clinically useful is based on whether the pain is arising from superficial, deep somatic, or visceral structures, or from damage to the nerves themselves. The latter pain problem is often referred to as 'neuropathic' pain. A thorough pain assessment, as described above, will usually permit characterisation of each pain into one of the following groups.

Superficial Pain

Superficial pain is caused by damage to cutaneous tissues and to the mucous membranes, for example, in the mouth. The simplest way to mimic superficial pain is to prick the skin with a pin. The pain has a sharp stinging quality which is well localised. This is due to the transmission of the pain signals by small-diameter myelinated nerve fibres. Superficial pain is often associated with the clinical signs of inflammation, such as redness, swelling and heat at the site of the pain. Prostaglandins, bradykinins and a variety of other chemical mediators play an important role in generating the pain.

Causes

Cancer is rarely directly responsible for superficial pain. Subcutaneous metastases do occur with some cancers such as melanoma, but do not usually cause pain. Occasionally, malignant subcutaneous nodules will become exquisitely tender even though there is no obvious inflammation or ulceration. The patient will be unable to lie on the nodules or bear anything (even clothes) from touching them. Local recurrence of breast cancer may lead to large numbers of nodules which become confluent and ulcerate the skin. The nodules may not be painful, but secondary infection will cause superficial pain, associated with an offensive discharge. Secondary infection can also play a role in exacerbating the pain of head and neck cancers which ulcerate through into the mouth. Superficial thrombophlebitis is associated classically with pancreatic cancer but also with other solid tumours, and may cause multiple painful lesions.

The commonest cause of superficial pain is skin damage from pressure. Most patients with advanced cancer become weak and bed-bound. If attention is not paid to pressure relief, skin redness is followed by ulceration over the pressure points of the body: the sacrum, greater trochanters, heels, thoracic spinous processes and the occiput. The earliest sign of damage to a pressure area is erythema which does not fade when the pressure is relieved. Superficial abrasion of the skin is the next stage and this is the most painful. Deeper ulcers cause less pain but are still distressing.

Cancer treatments can contribute to superficial pain. Mucositis is a painful side-effect of some chemotherapy agents and bone marrow transplantation. The mouth is usually affected by multiple small ulcers. Rarely, ulceration may be so extensive and painful that the patient is unable to eat or drink. Secondary fungal and bacterial infections may compound the problem, and delay healing. Mucositis may be associated with herpetic infection in some instances. Radiation therapy can also cause mucositis of the mouth, oesophagus, vagina and rectum if these organs are in the treatment field. Skin reactions with redness and desquamation can occur. If pain does develop, it usually begins several days after the start of treatment.

Treatment

Painful malignant nodules should be locally excised if possible. Radiotherapy may also be helpful for single nodules and for relatively small confluent areas of local recurrence. However, these treatments are of limited use if there are multiple discrete nodules. Some patients with breast cancer benefit from hormone therapy or chemotherapy. Other cancers may respond to specific regimens, for example, dacarbazine for melanoma. Whenever infection is complicating tumour fungation and is contributing to pain, appropriate antibiotics should be given.

Pharmacological treatments should be used to control pain while the effects of anti-cancer treatments are awaited or when the cancer cannot be directly controlled. The 'simple' analgesics, from step one of the WHO analgesic stepladder, offer the logical starting point. Paracetamol is cheap and safe. The usual dose is 1000 mg regularly every six hours. It is not contraindicated if liver secondaries are present but should be used cautiously in elderly people and patients with liver dysfunction. It is available in a number of formulations including tablets, capsules, elixir and suppositories. The tablets are large and may be difficult to swallow. The elixir can be more suitable although some preparations have an unpleasant taste. Unfortunately, paracetamol has limited effectiveness and other options are usually necessary.

NSAIDs have the theoretical advantage of treating the inflammation which commonly accompanies superficial pain. There are a wide variety of preparations and the choice depends on cost and convenience to the patient. Ideally, treatment should be once daily and the tablets should be small and coated so that they are easy to swallow. There is some evidence that a trial of another NSAID may be effective if partial relief is not obtained after two or three days (Day and Brooks, 1987). Increasing the dose of an NSAID beyond recommended levels does not increase the analgesic effect but does increase the incidence of side-effects. The combination of paracetamol and an NSAID is more effective than either used alone. If an NSAID has been effective, it should be continued as suppositories or injections when the patient becomes too weak to swallow tablets. NSAIDs should always be used cautiously in the elderly, patients with renal or liver impairment, bleeding diathesis, or peptic ulcer. Patients with advanced cancer are more likely to have peptic ulceration than the normal population. When prescribing NSAIDs, most doctors also prescribe cytoprotective agents which have been shown to reduce the risk of gastrointestinal haemorrhage or perforation in other patient groups receiving NSAIDs. Misoprostol protects against gastric, as well as duodenal, ulcers.

With superficial pain from a small number of subcutaneous nodules or ulcers, a topical NSAID preparation may be effective. The gel can be gently applied and then covered with plastic film or a dressing. Another useful topical analgesic cream is the eutectic mixture of local anaesthetics (EMLA) which contains lignocaine and prilocaine. This can also be applied under the protection of a plastic film and can give many hours of relief. Unfortunately, some patients develop skin reactions which necessitate stopping the treatment. An exciting but expensive new treatment for painful skin ulceration is the use of thermo-reversible gels. These gels are liquid when kept in a freezer but solidify when warmed. Upon contact with a malignant ulcer, the gel conforms to the surface of the ulcer before setting to produce a plastic-like coating. Local anaesthetics can be mixed with the gel to improve the analgesic effect. The rubifacient creams such as capsaicin rely on counter-irritation for pain relief. They often make superficial pain worse.

While the above measures can be used for painful pressure areas, prevention is the best form of management. Frequent turning of very weak patients and the use of pressure-relieving mattresses and aids can minimise the need for analgesics. If a painful ulcer does develop, topical NSAIDs can be very effective. Antibiotics may be necessary but patients are often too ill to take oral medications. The cachexia process, which is the usual cause of the weakness, prevents ulcer healing; only rarely is this a feasible objective.

Prevention is also the best way of managing painful mucositis. Good mouth care with frequent antiseptic mouth washes and regular prophylactic use of antifungal agents will minimise ulceration. Topical NSAID, steroid and local anaesthetic preparations may be used for established painful ulcers. Rarely, oral morphine may be necessary. Some patients benefit from a trial of acyclovir therapy for herpes infection.

Deep Somatic Pain

Deep somatic structures include muscle and bone. Pain arising in these organs is transmitted by larger unmyelinated nerve fibres. It is usually described as dull and aching. The pain is relatively well localised but spreads across a wider area than superficial pain. In some instances, deep pain is referred. For example, metastatic involvement of the neck of the femur or acetabulum may be felt in the knee. Tenderness may occur over the site of deep pain but signs of inflammation are rare, unless superficial spread of the cancer has also occurred. This frequently happens with head and neck cancers, which may arise superficially, but quickly spread into the subjacent muscle and bone.

Causes

Skeletal metastases occur frequently. Between 30% and 70% of cancer patients will develop spread to bone. The commonly listed primary sites for bone metastases are lung, breast, kidney, prostate and thyroid. Myeloma is also associated with bone involvement. Less commonly, bone metastases occur with colorectal, pancreatic, cervical and ovarian cancers. The usual site for metastases is the vertebral bodies, followed by pelvis, femurs, ribs, skull and humeri. Metastases cause bone destruction which eventually leads to bone fracture or collapse. Back or neck pain should prompt a review of spinal cord function to exclude evidence of cord compression.

Any patient presenting with pain over the skeleton should be investigated. X-rays of the painful site may reveal bone destruction (osteolysis), new bone formation (osteoblastic metastases), a mixed picture, or they may appear normal. Osteoblastic metastases occur with prostate and breast cancer. Bone scintigraphy uses radioactive tracers to label areas of bone reaction. Metastases usually cause increased activity in the bone and may show up before they can be seen on radiographs. If a bone scintiscan shows potential metastases in the femurs and other long bones which are not associated with symptoms, radiographic examination should be undertaken to exclude impending fracture. Metastases may also be seen on CT and MRI scans. The former can be helpful in detecting acetabular metastases that do not show on pelvic x-rays and metastases in the base of the skull. MRI scans can detect intramedullary spread where the cancer spreads within the marrow and does not cause bone changes.

Lymph node metastases in the groins, axillae and neck will cause pain if they become large enough. Retroperitoneal lymph node metastases produce a dull aching back pain. Other less common causes of deep somatic pain include soft tissue and muscle infiltration (usually by head and neck cancers, lung cancers and mesotheliomas), and sarcomas. Raised intracranial pressure is caused by primary or metastatic brain tumours. Secondary hydrocephalus or cystic degeneration of a tumour post-treatment may mimic the effects of a brain tumour. The resultant headache is caused by tension on the falx and the meninges. Meningeal deposits also produce an unpleasant headache.

The most common non-malignant condition which causes deep somatic pain, given the age of most cancer patients, is arthritis. Patients recovering from major cancer surgery may experience deep somatic pain for several days despite successful removal of the cancer. Rarely, post-operative patients will develop deep-seated abscesses which produce constant pain as well as many of the other features of advanced cancer such as anorexia, weakness and weight loss. Localised inflammatory changes may not be apparent, at least until the abscess tracks more superficially. Fevers, rigors and sweats help to distinguish this treatable non-malignant cause of pain. Some patients develop deep venous thrombosis or gross lymphoedema which produce painful swollen limbs.

Treatment

Bone pain from metastatic cancer will often respond to radiotherapy. In some patients, the pain relief may be almost immediate, well before any anticipated effect on the size of the cancer. This observation has led to the use of shorter courses of radiotherapy for bone pain. Some centres give a single dose which is repeated if the pain returns. This is particularly helpful for patients who already have advanced disease and for whom travelling for treatment will further deplete dwindling reserves of energy. If bone fracture or collapse has produced mechanical instability, radiotherapy may produce minimal analgesia.

For pharmacological treatment, patients should be started on paracetamol and then an NSAID, as described for superficial pain. If the pain is not controlled, the next step is to use a weak opioid in combination with the simple analgesics. A widely used weak opioid is dextropropoxyphene which is available in tablets combined with paracetamol. The usual dose is equivalent to 1000 mg paracetamol and 100 mg dextropropoxyphene every 4–6 h. Some accumulation of dextropropoxyphene occurs and 24 h should be allowed to reach steady state before it is dismissed as ineffective. Codeine and dihydrocodeine are also widely used. The usual dose is 30–60 mg codeine four hourly, much more than the dose of codeine that is contained in many combination analgesics available over-the-counter from retail pharmacies. The slow-release preparations of dihydrocodeine are more convenient because of the 12-hourly dosing frequency. Tramadol is another weak opioid that has recently become available in the UK. Experience suggests that it is more potent than the other weak opioids. This may reflect other non-opioid actions of tramadol. It must be given four hourly. The side-effects of all weak opioids include confusion, drowsiness, constipation and nausea. These side-effects are more common in the elderly. The management of these side-effects is the same as for morphine and is described below. Given that weak opioids are rarely sufficient to control cancer pain, many palliative-care doctors leave out this step. It can be helpful to use weak opioids for patients who are very afraid of starting morphine. This offers time to explore the issues and fears while still treating the pain.

The next step is the use of strong opioids. Eventually, strong opioids are required for most patients with cancer pain. Morphine is the strong opioid of choice. It is widely available and its use has been thoroughly documented. The pharmacology of morphine has been extensively revised in the last decade. Previously, it was thought that free morphine was the active drug. Morphine was known to be metabolised by glucuronidation, mostly in the liver, but the metabolites were thought to be inactive. The development of an assay system that could distinguish free morphine from the metabolites revealed the importance of one of the metabolites, morphine-6-glucuronide (M6G). When morphine passes through the liver, it is converted to large quantities of morphine-3-glucuronide (M3G), which is inactive, and smaller quantities of M6G. M6G is at least 10 times more potent as an analgesic than free morphine when given intravenously. The analgesic effect of morphine is therefore a combination of the effects of free morphine and M6G. Because M6G is excreted via the kidneys, accumulation may occur if a patient has renal impairment.

Morphine is usually given orally, starting with a dose of 10 mg morphine elixir or immediate release tablets four hourly. Lower starting doses (2.5–5 mg) should be used for elderly patients, patients with severely impaired liver function, or patients who are very frightened of starting morphine despite reassurance. Chronic obstructive respiratory disease is not a contraindication for starting oral morphine but the lower dose is usually appropriate for this group as well. The usual dosing frequency of four hourly should be extended for patients with moderate to severe renal and severe liver impairment (not just liver metastases). These patients, who are often elderly, may only require 6-, 8- or even 12-hourly dosing depending on the duration of the analgesic effect.

As with the weak opioids, some dose accumulation occurs when morphine is first started. This means that an increase in the regular background dose of morphine should only be considered if the pain is not relieved after 24 h. This allows time for the morphine levels to reach steady state. Longer intervals between dose measures, up to three or four days, should be considered for patients with renal and liver impairment, and for the elderly. When a dose increment is made, there should be a 30%–50% increase. There is no maximum dose. Each patient must have the dose individually titrated upwards until the pain is relieved. Rarely, some patients may require more than 1000 mg of morphine per day.

Most cancer pain is chronic and continuous. However, there are two important patterns of intermittent pain which should be distinguished because their management is different:

1. Break-through pain occurs before the next regular dose of analgesia is due. It usually means that the regular dose is inadequate and the levels of analgesic are too low. An extra dose of morphine, equivalent to the regular four-hourly dose, can be given when pain occurs. If sufficient time has passed for the regular morphine dose to have reached steady-state, the regular morphine dose can be increased.
2. Incident pain is pain which occurs with movement, weight bearing, a change of a surgical dressing or some other specific incident. The patient is usually pain-free at rest. The regular morphine dose should not be increased because this will render the patient drowsy at rest. A better strategy is to give a four-hourly equivalent dose of morphine 30 min before the incident which causes the pain. Alternatives such as dextromoramide 5–20 mg, given 15 min before the percipient or patient self-administration of nitrous oxide/oxygen mixture at the time of the incident, can be considered. Another option is sublingual fentanyl or sufentanil 3–5 min before the

incident. A surgically correctable lesion such as impending or actual bone fracture should always be excluded as a cause of incident pain.

There are now a variety of slow-release morphine preparations which can be used when the patient's morphine requirements have been titrated to steady-state. Converting to these preparations is achieved by calculating the total daily morphine dosage and dividing by the daily dosing frequency of the new preparation, halving the total dose for 12-hourly preparations or using the total dose for daily preparations. These formulations should not be used for break-through or incident pain.

Although most patients will only require oral medications, alternative routes need to be used if the patient cannot tolerate this route. Some of the indications for changing the route of administration include persistent nausea and vomiting from inoperable bowel obstruction, for example, inability to swallow oral medications such as occurs with oesophageal obstruction, and altered conscious level when the patient is dying. The rectal route requires an equivalent dose to the oral. Suppositories can be given four hourly or the slow-release tablets can be given 12 hourly. This route has largely been surpassed by subcutaneous administration. There is no need to use the intramuscular route; it causes more discomfort and the levels of morphine and M6G are no different. Diamorphine is used most often in the UK because of the high solubility. This allows for high doses to be delivered in low volumes. The equivalent dose is 30% of the oral dose. It can be given four hourly by intermittent injection through a butterfly needle or small-bore cannula that is left subcutaneously. More often, a portable syringe driver is used to infuse the opioid continuously. In countries where diamorphine is not available, alternatives such as morphine and hydromorphone are used. When high concentrations of morphine are required, the morphine tartrate salt can be used, although it is not as soluble as diamorphine. The epidural and intrathecal route are rarely used, usually if appropriate doses of opioids and other analgesics cause unacceptable side-effects when given by other routes. It requires experienced personnel to insert the cannulae and administer the drugs. Failure of oral morphine to relieve pain is not an indication for epidural morphine.

Management of Opioid Side-Effects
The most feared side-effect of morphine therapy is respiratory depression. This is extremely rare when oral morphine is titrated in the manner described. Pain serves as the 'antidote' to this potential effect of morphine. Oral morphine can even be used in patients with pre-existing chronic obstructive respiratory disease who also have cancer pain. Once the patient has been on morphine for more than a few days, the respiratory centre becomes tolerant to morphine. If the patient takes an accidental overdose of morphine, drowsiness will occur but the patient will not stop breathing. Naloxone should only be used with extreme caution to reverse the drowsiness because it will precipitate severe pain and agitation. It is usually better to allow the effects of the morphine to subside gradually as it is metabolised. Respiratory depression may occur when severe pain controlled by morphine is then relieved by some other means such as nerve block. This can be avoided by converting patients from slow-release morphine preparations to

immediate release morphine given four hourly prior to the procedure, then lowering the morphine dose if the procedure is effective.

Another common fear is the fear of addiction. Physical dependence does occur when people take morphine for more than one or two weeks. If the morphine is stopped suddenly, the patient will experience anxiety, irritability, chills, sweating, cramping abdominal pain and diarrhoea. Usually, the patient will experience severe pain and distress before these other symptoms develop. These behaviours are not to be confused with psychological addiction. Cancer patients who take morphine for pain do not develop psychological dependency (Schug et al 1992). If a cancer patient has a pre-existing drug dependency problem, morphine should still be used, but the patient should be managed in collaboration with a specialised drug-dependency team.

The idea of morphine addiction was often linked to the phenomenon of tolerance. Tolerance is characterised by escalating morphine doses in order to maintain pain control. Concern about this problem often led doctors to delay starting morphine so that it would not lose its effect when the patient was dying. In practice, tolerance is not an issue. When the morphine dose has been titrated to control the pain, most patients then have a stable dose requirement. There is no evidence that the metabolism of morphine increases with time. If the pain increases, this is usually a sign of disease progression and an indication to increase the dose of morphine. Sometimes, patients increase the dose of morphine for its anxiolytic effect, often at night. Unlike the effect on pain, the effect of morphine on fear is short-lived and tolerance does develop. Prompt recognition of this problem will allow psychological support and more effective anxiolytic therapy.

Drowsiness is an important side-effect that occurs when patients first start morphine therapy. Patients should be warned of the possibility but advised that the effect usually wears off after two or three days. If a patient is very worried by this, a smaller starting dose can be used (2.5 mg four hourly). The low dose may not relieve the pain but patients are more worried by the possibility of drowsiness than they are of the pain. If drowsiness persists after a patient has been on a stable dose of morphine for more than three days and the patient is still physically well, the dose of morphine should be lowered by 25%. Provided that the pain remains controlled, the drowsiness will subside. However, if pain recurs and a balance cannot be struck between pain relief and drowsiness, an alternative opioid (see below) or some other analgesic strategy such as neural blockade should be tried. Patients who are dying become drowsy as part of the disease process. Their drowsiness should not be attributed to morphine. Lowering or stopping the dose of morphine in these patients will cause extreme distress. More often it is the family who are worried by the change and they need simple reassurance that the morphine is not responsible.

Nausea and vomiting may occur in 50% of patients who start oral morphine. A regular anti-emetic should be started at the same time as the morphine: haloperidol 1.5 mg once or twice daily, metoclopramide 10 mg six hourly, or cyclizine 50 mg eight hourly. Morphine-induced nausea is usually temporary. The anti-emetics can often be reviewed and stopped after three to four days. If nausea and vomiting occurs weeks or months after starting morphine, some other cause, such as hypercalcaemia or constipation, will be responsible.

Constipation is universal with opioids. A bowel softener and stimulant should always be prescribed with regular morphine unless there are specific contra-indications such as bowel obstruction. A softening laxative such as lactulose given alone is often inadequate.

Less common side-effects of morphine include bronchospasm, itch and urinary retention. The latter usually occurs when morphine is given intra-spinally. Some patients experience confusion and hallucinations associated with other excitatory manifestations such as myoclonus. These effects may be dose-related, responding to a reduction in the morphine dose. Changing to another strong opioid is often more effective because of incomplete cross-tolerance.

Alternative Strong Opioids

There are several alternative strong opioids. The choice varies from country to country. Methadone is one of the cheapest and most widely available options. It is a difficult drug to use because of its very variable half-life. Methadone is best started with loading doses (2.5–5 mg for opioid naive patients) given at 30 minute intervals until the pain is relieved. The patient then waits until the pain begins to return before taking repeat doses until the pain is relieved again. This process is repeated whenever the pain starts to recur. Over a two-week period, a regular pattern of methadone usage will emerge which will guide prescribing. Phenazocine is another alternative which has the advantage of an eight-hourly dosing interval. However, the fixed-dose tablets limit its usefulness when large doses are required. Oxycodone can be given rectally but this is rarely a desirable feature. More recently, fentanyl transdermal patches have been developed. The patches provide a relatively constant level of fentanyl over a 2–3 day period. This reduces the number of tablets taken by the patient, although some form of 'rescue' analgesia, such as oral morphine, is needed for break-through pain. The patches are very expensive and should only be considered when the oral route is unavailable. Pethidine and pentazocine must not be used as alternatives to morphine. They have no place in the management of cancer pain.

Whenever a strong opioid is prescribed, time should be spent with the patient and family eliciting their fears and reassuring them. They are usually worried about the traditional myths surrounding the use of morphine: addiction, prema-ture death and the risk of unrelieved pain when the patient is dying if morphine is used too soon. It is often helpful to mention the possibility of morphine therapy when simple analgesics are first prescribed. This encourages the fears to surface before the morphine is actually needed. Careful explanations should be given about how the morphine is to be used and written down. Patients and families will be reassured to know that extra doses of morphine can be given for break-through and incident pain without risk of overdosage.

Other Treatments for Deep Somatic Pain

There are several other options for managing specific types of deep somatic pain. Surgical stabilisation will relieve the pain of impending or actual pathological fractures, as well as preserve function. Even patients with very advanced disease may benefit from fixation of a fractured neck of femur. Procedures are available for unstable pathological fractures of vertebrae. However, these procedures are technically difficult and require a patient who is well enough to withstand a major operation.

Bisphosphanates are being used to treat bone pain. Infusions of 60–120 mg have been given at fortnightly and monthly intervals with good effect in some patients with myeloma, breast cancer and prostate cancer. Calcitonin injections are also effective for bone pain but the frequency of administration (six hourly) limit its use. Radioactive pharmaceutical agents have been developed which concentrate in the marrow at the sites of metastatic cancer and deliver a short-range dose of radiation. They are useful for widespread bone involvement, for example with prostate cancer, but there is transient suppression of marrow function. Transphenoidal pituitary ablation has been used as an analgesic in the past. It is an effective technique even with tumours that are not hormonally responsive. However, there are significant risks including damage to the optic chiasma and the improved use of other analgesics has obviated its use.

Opioids can be used for the headache caused by raised intracranial pressure, indeed they become the only option when a patient is dying and unable to swallow tablets. However, steroids are more effective. The conventional maximal dose is 16 mg of dexamethasone, but higher doses, up to 100 mg, can be used if the patient feels that the quality of life achieved is worthwhile. Dexamethasone can be given by subcutaneous injection if the patient is unable to swallow, for example, because of a brain-stem glioma.

Deep-seated infections associated with cancer can often be successfully managed with prolonged courses of oral antibiotics if surgical drainage is not feasible. Rotating courses of clindamycin and augmentin are easily tolerated and give the necessary anaerobic cover. A significant improvement in quality of life can often be achieved, the patient may seemingly 'resurrect' from what was thought to be a terminal decline.

Neural blockade techniques (nerve blocks) were widely used before the pharmacological treatments became better known. Most blocks have a limited duration of effect, usually less than two months, despite the fact that nerves are damaged to achieve analgesia. Neurolysis is achieved with compounds such as phenol, with surgical resection, or by applying intense heat or cold. There is the associated risk of damage to motor nerve function. Nerve blocks still have a role in selected cases, for example, when patients cannot tolerate or do not want to take oral medications. There are blocks which can be used for pain from head and neck cancers, but they are technically difficult. The brachial plexus can be blocked for arm pain but the results are poor and the risks of arm weakness very high. Paravertebral blocks are used for chest-wall pain, blocking the intercostal nerves at, above and below the level of the pain. Surgery can also be used to achieve the same result. Recently, some success has been achieved by infusing bupivacaine into the pleural cavity. A psoas compartment block, where a catheter is inserted just beneath the psoas fascia, can provide effective analgesia for a fractured neck of femur when an operation is not possible. A cordotomy can be used to disrupt the spinothalamic tract in the cervical spinal cord. This produces dissociated anaesthesia with relief of pain on the contralateral side. It can be done as an open surgical or a closed percutaneous procedure, but should only be considered for patients with unilateral pain, preferably below the umbilicus.

Visceral Pain

Visceral pain arises from the visceral organs in the peritoneal cavity and the mediastinum. Like deep somatic pain, it usually has a dull aching quality. When solid organs are involved, the pain is constant in nature. Hollow organs, such as the bowel and bladder, usually produce intermittent pain, for example, bowel colic and bladder spasms. Visceral pain is not as well localised as superficial pain but is often felt in the general anatomical area of the involved organ. Examples include pain in the right upper quadrant of the abdomen from liver enlargement, low abdominal pain with pelvic disease and epigastric discomfort from pancreatic cancer. Small bowel colic is felt in the periumbilical region and pain from the large bowel may be felt in the left lower quadrant, suprapubic region, or the right lower quadrant.

Causes

Malignant causes of visceral pain are common. Liver metastases occur with colorectal, breast, lung and a variety of other cancers. The pain is due to the stretching of the liver capsule rather than the metastases per se. Slowly growing lesions may produce gross hepatomegaly without pain – a sudden bleed into a small metastasis can cause severe pain. Pelvic tumours are usually primary, arising from the rectum or pelvic organs. Metastases can occur in the pelvis from transcoelomic spread. Splenomegaly occurs with the haematological malignancies and is often relatively painless until the spleen is very enlarged or until splenic infarction occurs. Lung metastases are painless but mediastinal involvement may cause a deep aching chest pain. Malignant involvement of the bowel by direct infiltration or malignant adhesions causes colic. Infiltration of the bladder results in bladder spasms. Surprisingly, malignant obstructions of the ureters and biliary tract rarely cause pain.

Non-malignant causes of visceral pain are infrequent in cancer patients. Some people will have pre-existing conditions such as angina pectoris. Abscess formation should be considered if there are systemic symptoms suggesting infection. The effects of prior radiation to the abdomen or post-operative non-malignant adhesions should always be considered when patients develop pain and other signs of bowel obstruction.

Treatment

Surgical and other anti-cancer options should be considered for malignant causes of visceral pain. New treatments are being developed for treating liver metastases, for example. Resection of isolated colorectal metastases may even result in cure. Techniques such as hepatic artery infusion of chemotherapeutic agents and the use of cryotherapy for multiple lesions are available in some specialist centres. For bowel obstruction, useful palliation of pain may be achieved if an obstructing tumour is surgically bypassed even if resection is not possible.

Pharmacological measures are needed for patients with progressive disease. The simple analgesics should be tried initially but opioids are usually required. Morphine is often effective as a single analgesic for the pain of liver metastases. Steroids may be helpful for painful hepatomegaly. Specific analgesics may be necessary for certain pains: anticholinergics such as hyoscine for bowel colic and oxybutynin for bladder spasms.

Nerve blocks have a limited role, particularly for those patients who are intolerant of oral medications. Coeliac plexus blockade can relieve pain in the liver, pancreas and proximal intestine. It requires an experienced practitioner using radioimaging to guide to the needle. An effective block may last many months. Hypotension is an immediate side-effect but this is usually transient. Diarrhoea may occur, but this is controllable. Lumbar sympathectomy may be helpful for bladder spasms. Hypogastric blocks are technically very difficult but have been used for pelvic pain.

Neuropathic Pain

Neuropathic pain (nerve pain) is caused by damage to nerves: peripheral, autonomic or central. It occurs in up to one third of patients with cancer and is one of the most difficult types of pain to control. Nerve pain is frequently not recognised. Even when the diagnosis is made, appropriate treatments are often not used. Patients may have experienced escalating pain for many months before effective treatment is offered.

Nerve pain is variously described by patients as burning, stabbing, shooting, like 'electric shocks' or 'pins and needles'. It is often the cause of pain which radiates into a limb or around the trunk. Examination will reveal evidence of nerve damage in the area of the pain. Sensation will be reduced or heightened. Sometimes, lightly stroking the skin will trigger pain, a phenomenon known as *allodynia*. Motor function will also be reduced if the nerve damage is extensive enough, along with reduced reflexes. If autonomic dysfunction occurs, the painful area appears red and swollen, and feels warmer than normal. Some nerve pains are not associated with any signs. Coeliac plexus involvement will cause a gnawing, burning back pain. Infiltration or irritation of the rectum produces tenesmus, which is a very unpleasant feeling that the bowels need to move.

Causes

Nerve pain is commonly caused by cancer directly compressing and damaging nerves. Head and neck cancers will cause pain radiating to the top of the head, into the ear, or down into the neck. Brachial plexus lesions occur with breast and lung cancers, causing pain in the arm and weakness. Vertebral body collapse, extradural masses and spinal cord compression can all cause nerve pain radiating around the dermatomes that are directly damaged, and sometimes down into the legs as well. Chest-wall involvement by lung cancers and meso-theliomas frequently have a mixture of deep somatic pain and evidence of intercostal nerve damage. The lumbosacral plexus will be affected by cancers of the bowel, cervix and kidney. The last mentioned causes pain which radiates into the groin on the affected side. Pancreatic cancer often damages the coeliac plexus, and tenesmus is associated with rectal carcinomas. Rarely, brain metas-tases which cause hemiparesis may also cause nerve pain.

Surgery can cause nerve damage. Chest-wall pain sometimes occurs post-mastectomy and post-thoracotomy. Abdomino–perineal resections for rectal cancer may produce sacral and perineal pain. The history must be used to distinguish from a post-surgical cause from cancer recurrence. With the former, the pain will have been present from the time of the operation; with the latter, the pain will start several months later. Investigations may be unreliable because post-operative scarring distorts the architecture and limits the size of the re-currence. Too often, patients with recurrent disease have been repeatedly reassured despite worsening pain. A high index of suspicion is needed until the diagnosis is confirmed to ensure that adequate analgesic treatment is started.

Nerve damage can result from the delayed effects of radiotherapy. Fortunately, this is very uncommon but some patients given local radiotherapy post-mastectomy may present many years later with a brachial plexopathy. As with surgical scarring, the fibrosis induced by radiotherapy poses a difficult diagnostic problem. The most common non-malignant cause of nerve pain is shingles. The acute pain often subsides as the lesions heal, to be replaced by the burning dysaethesia of post-herpetic neuralgia.

Treatment

Anti-cancer treatments can be less effective for nerve pain. If nerves have been infiltrated, the possibility of curative resection is reduced. Radiotherapy and chemotherapy can relieve nerve pain, but their efficacy is reduced if there is fibrosis associated with the malignant process. Usually, any beneficial effect on nerve pain is more short-lived than for other types of pain.

There are a wide range of drug therapies recommended for nerve pain but the most effective combination has to be determined for each individual patient. The simple analgesics and the opioids should be started first. However, nerve pain is rarely contained by morphine. When morphine is first started, the pain will improve but it often returns within a short time. Increasing doses of morphine continue to improve the pain temporarily but total relief is unusual and the pain keeps recurring. Other analgesics should be added to improve the quality and duration of analgesia. Antidepressants have an analgesic effect which is indepen-dent of the antidepressant effect. Patients with advanced cancer are more sensitive to the side-effects of the tricyclic group. Amitriptyline should therefore be started at 10–25 mg and increased by the same dose every two or three days until the pain is relieved or side-effects, such as drowsiness and dry mouth, occur. The newer selective antidepressants do not appear to be as effective.

Several anticonvulsants are effective for nerve pain, including carbamazepine, sodium valproate and clonazepam. The choice of anticonvulsant will depend on the preference of the doctor. There is some evidence that clonazepam is more effective (Swerdlow and Cundhill, 1981) and less likely to cause side-effects. Whichever drug is used, the initial dose should be kept low and then built up gradually, as for amitriptyline, to minimise drowsiness. Steroids have been recommended on the basis that they reduce perineural oedema. They are also helpful for other symptoms of cancer, particularly nausea and anorexia. Recent interest has centred on the membrane-stabilising antiarrhythmic drugs including flecainide, mexilitine and tocainide. These drugs are used in their normal cardiac dosages and cause fewer side-effects. For example, flecainide is usually started at a dose of 100 mg but can be increased to 200 mg b.d.

Topical local anaesthetics such as EMLA cream are useful for patients who have allodynia. They can be applied then covered with plastic film. Lignocaine can be given as a slow intravenous bolus in a dose of 3 mg/kg over five minutes. The analgesic effect occurs within minutes, making it a useful treatment for severe pain in a patient who cannot take oral medications. The effect can be sustained with a continuous infusion of subcutaneous lignocaine at 2–4 mg per minute. Ketamine has been effective in patients with nerve pain unresponsive to other options. A low starting dose of 10 mg followed by an infusion of 10–15 mg per hour avoids the usual psychotropic effects of ketamine. It can be given orally in doses of 25–50 mg 4-6-hourly. Local skin reactions may limit how long the ketamine can be used for.

Neural blockade techniques run the risk of making nerve pain worse by increasing the amount of nerve damage. Many of the procedures described for treating deep somatic pain are used for nerve pain. In addition, sacral nerve pain can be treated with a caudal injection of phenol. Loss of bladder and bowel continence will occur, but many patients with advanced pelvic cancers already have a colostomy and a urinary catheter. The epidural route is useful for infusing local anaesthetics as well as morphine into the epidural space. When the local anaesthetic is titrated carefully, motor function can be preserved. The epidural catheter can be tunnelled subcutaneously. Infection is a potential risk but rarely prevents catheters from being left in place for more than six months

Summary

By following the above recommendations, pain control should be achieved in more than 90% of patients. For the remainder, successful pain management will require the expertise of pain specialists and palliative-care physicians. Whenever pain is not controlled, practitioners should never hesitate to ask for advice. Even if a specialist service is not readily available, there are numerous hospice programmes which will provide advice over the telephone. Early referral should be considered for patients with multiple distressing symptoms, severe emotional and family distress, and existing drug dependency problems.

3 – Management of Respiratory Symptoms

Introduction

The major respiratory symptoms associated with advanced cancer include breathlessness, cough and haemoptysis. These symptoms occur with primary lung cancers, metastatic disease to the lungs and in association with other conditions.

Breathlessness

Breathlessness is a subjective experience characterised by difficulty in breathing. Patients will describe two types of difficulty: limited exercise capacity and a feeling of distress. This distinction has implications for symptomatic treatment. If a patient has difficulty getting from the bed to the toilet, for example, medications which have an anxiolytic effect, but do not improve exercise tolerance, will not be helpful. The patient will feel sedated but still not be able to get from the bed to the toilet.

There are several mechanisms which produce the sensation of breathlessness. It is likely that discrepancies between respiratory demand and effort are monitored centrally from signals generated in respiratory muscle fibres and muscle spindles. Muscle fatigue, particularly diaphragmatic, may also play a role. The cachexia syndrome affects the diaphragm as well as other muscle groups. In animal models, receptors exist within the lungs which signal changes in pressure and volume. These 'J' receptors may be responsible for breathlessness associated with lymphangitis and other intrapulmonary causes of dyspnoea.

Hypoxia probably does not play a major role in causing breathlessness. Most breathless patients with advanced cancer are not hypoxaemic. Furthermore, rendering severely hypoxaemic does not cause dyspnoea. The role of oxygen in treating breathlessness will be considered later.

Other factors, such as fear, depression and anxiety, can aggravate breathlessness. The distress associated with breathlessness can be extreme. The need to breath is fundamental to life. Any perceived difficulty will cause a fear of choking and suffocation. Characteristically, patients will lie awake at night lest they stop breathing on falling asleep.

Anxiety may be a cause of breathlessness, usually as a trigger of the hyperventilation syndrome. There are some cancer patients who experience paroxysms of breathlessness associated with the tingling and faintness which characterise the syndrome. However, it is unwise to attribute breathlessness solely to anxiety even if hyperventilation reproduces the symptoms. Some physical causes of dyspnoea may produce high levels of anxiety out of proportion to the physical signs. Mediastinal disease with early tracheal compression is one example.

The estimated prevalence of breathlessness varies considerably. It becomes more common with advancing disease with up to 75% of lung cancer patients experiencing dyspnoea in some studies. Dyspnoea is less likely with other diagnoses. Men are more likely to be affected than women. Progressive dyspnoea is associated with a poor prognosis.

Breathlessness is also very distressing to carers, professionals and families alike. Many carers rate dyspnoea as more distressing than pain, even though it occurs less frequently. It is important to maintain the patient's perspective as the guide to treatment! Carers sometimes misinterpret the physical signs of increased respiratory rate (tachypnoea) and depth (hyperpnoea) as breathlessness. Support for staff will be needed when patients underplay symptoms or refuse medications.

Physical Causes of Breathlessness

Cancer-Related Causes

Lung cancers frequently produce breathlessness by causing obstruction to bronchi, less commonly by narrowing the trachea. When collapse of lung tissue occurs distally, ventilation–perfusion mismatch occurs. Direct extension into lung parenchyma and intra-alveolar spread may also produce dyspnoea.

Lung metastases may be asymptomatic, even when multiple. However, breathlessness will occur if external bronchial compression occurs. Lymphangitis carcinomatosa can occur with lung, prostate, breast and gastrointestinal cancers. Widespread lymphatic obstruction results in severe dyspnoea and characteristic x-ray findings.

Pleural disease occurs with mesothelioma and secondary spread from lung, breast, melanoma, ovary and other cancers. Widespread pleural spread will cause restriction of the hemithorax. Pleural effusions usually reflect lymphatic obstruction rather than extent of pleural disease, but produce dyspnoea by the same mechanism of restriction. Rarely, extensive locally recurrent breast cancer will also produce a similar effect.

Malignant pericardial effusions may cause severe dyspnoea. The clinical features include pulsus paradoxus, positive Kussmant's sign, soft or absent heart sounds and hypertension. Chest x-ray, CT scanning and ECHO cardiography will help establish the diagnosis. Another correctable cause of dyspnoea is superior vena caval obstruction (SVCO).

Treatment-Related Causes

Some anti-cancer treatments will produce breathlessness. Lobectomy or pneumonectomy may leave some residual dyspnoea on exertion, but this is usually non-progressive. Radiotherapy to normal lung tissues may reduce a pneumonitis in up to 15% of patients. Breathlessness is the major symptom which usually occurs 2–3 months after treatment. Chest x-ray findings include alveolar shadowing and fibrotic thickening.

Several chemotherapy agents are known to cause lung damage. Bleomycin is the drug most commonly implicated. Risk factors, including age, prior radiation treatment, use of other drugs and oxygen therapy increase the possibility of pneumonitis.

Other Conditions

Chronic obstructive pulmonary disease and asthma are common causes of breathlessness in cancer patients. The association between these diseases, cigarette smoking and lung cancer is very high. It may be difficult to distinguish between the variable causes in any individual patient. Asthma tends to be episodic with wheezing during exacerbations. Stable levels of dyspnoea on exertion characterise chronic bronchitis and emphysema, but rapid deterioration may be due to acute bronchitis rather than the progression of cancer. Even when the breathlessness is not progressive, a trial of bronchodilator therapy and steroids may be warranted.

Acute-on-chronic bronchitis has been mentioned as an example of an infection causing dyspnoea. Pneumonias may occur in cancer patients. When bronchial obstruction is present, bacterial infection will persist until the airway is cleared. Often the infection will be anaerobic, causing systemic symptoms including fever and weight loss. However, breathlessness may be a prominent feature. Infections are an important complication in patients receiving chemotherapy. Early recognition and aggressive treatment are important.

Thromboembolic phenomena are generally more common in cancer patients. This propensity is increased when patients are treated with chemotherapy or when central venous access lines are present. Pulmonary emboli usually occur suddenly, although multiple small emboli may cause a more gradual increase in dyspnoea. Anxiety is a common association, haemoptysis and pleural chest pain are less so. Chest x-rays do not usually show effects of emboli.

Ischaemic heart disease is more common in the age group at risk of cancer. Some patients experience breathlessness as an 'angina-equivalent' in the absence of chest pain. The association with exercise, exposure to cold and abnormal ECG findings will often precede the diagnosis of cancer. Heart failure may occur in cancer patients giving rise to some diagnostic difficulties if pericardial tamponade is suspected.

Severe anaemia may cause dyspnoea. Usually, the haemoglobin level will be lower than 9.0 g/l. A history of blood loss may be present and pallor will be a prominent feature.

Assessment of Dyspnoea

Given the range of causes described above, a thorough history and clinical examination is indicated when assessing a breathless patient. Attention must be paid to the cardiovascular and other systems as well as the chest.

Respiratory function tests have a very limited role. Most breathless patients with advanced cancer have great difficulty in co-operating with even simple peak flow measures. A therapeutic trial without investigation is warranted in these situations. A chest x-ray is a simple investigation which can even be undertaken in the patient's home. Occasionally an ultrasound is helpful to confirm and localise an effusion.

Routine blood tests will confirm severe anaemia. Arterial blood gases are rarely indicated. Pulse oximetry has been a useful alternative in the clinical trials setting. Rarely, CT scanning, echocardiography, ventilation/perfusion, scintigraphy and pulmonary angiography may be indicated. Sudden deterioration of a patient undergoing treatment will require bronchoscopy and possible lung biopsy if the diagnosis is not clear.

For clinical trials, a variety of instruments are available to measure dyspnoea. Unfortunately, most have been developed for studying patients with non-malignant conditions. Cancer patients have difficulty filling out long and detailed questionnaires. Most studies have used a simple visual analogue scale or the Borg scale. The EORTC Quality of Life questionnaire has a lung cancer module suitable for conducting more detailed surveys.

Management of Dyspnoea

As with pain, the treatment of dyspnoea should not be withheld until investigations are complete.

Eliciting Attributions

Before embarking on treatment, some understanding should be gained about the patients' and families' fears. The anxiety is usually obvious and gently asking 'Are you afraid that you might suffocate/choke?' will often elicit the deepest fear. It is also helpful to ask 'Are you afraid to go to sleep?' Some patients are reassured by the explanation that their anxiety is a sign that the body is *not* ready to die. This explanation will be important if sedative drugs are being contemplated. Otherwise the patient will misinterpret the therapeutic effect and, paradoxically, will become worse. Another useful explanation is that the sensation of breathlessness does not mean that the person is running short of oxygen; most patients will have normal oxygen saturation levels. Breathlessness can be likened to a series of signals which from another organ would be registered as pain but from the lungs can only be registered as a sense of running out of air. This explanation can help explain the use of morphine.

Mention has already been made of the importance of recognising exercise limitation as the cause of a patient's distress. A higher priority would be given to those treatments which might improve exercise capacity.

Oncological Treatments

Wherever possible, treatment of breathlessness from cancer should be directed against the cancer. Some non-oncology specialists and general practitioners feel very pessimistic whenever a patient is diagnosed with cancer. Even if anti-cancer treatments have already been tried, further therapy may be possible.

Radiotherapy remains the most important anti-cancer option, particularly for patients with endobronchial obstruction. Recently, the trend has been to use short courses (one or two treatments), to minimise the effects of travelling for treatments. The concomitant use of steroids may be necessary if the patient has tracheal compression or SVCO. Some centres use brachytherapy to deliver high doses of radiation directly on to the cancer. This requires the use of an endo-bronchial catheter and an after-loading device to place the radioactive source accurately.

Chemotherapy has a limited role to play, particularly with non-small-cell carcinoma of the lung. Excellent palliation can be obtained with multi-agent chemotherapy in patients presenting with dyspnoea and limited-extent small-cell carcinoma. When patients have extensive disease, single-agent etoposide can provide good palliation with a minimum of side-effects. Hair loss is frequent, but systemic toxicity is more tolerable than more aggressive regimens. Patients with lung metastases tend to respond less well even if the primary disease is usually considered responsive to treatment, for example, breast cancer. Nevertheless, a trial of chemotherapy may be well worthwhile. The results of chemotherapy and hormone therapy usually take several weeks. Alternative means of controlling the dyspnoea should be used and then withdrawn if a response occurs.

Other options have been developed for specifically treating endobronchial lesions. High-energy laser beams can be aimed at tumours during bronchoscopy. This will cause immediate tissue destruction, reopening the lumen and thereby improving symptoms. The treatment can be repeated at intervals but the require-ment for bronchoscopy and the cost are limiting factors. Cryotherapy has been used as an alternative to laser therapy.

Stents have been used to maintain patency of bronchi. An expandable wire stent or a silastic tube can be placed during bronchoscopy. The complication rate is relatively high, with up to 10% mortality being reported due to infection or haemorrhage. Tumours may grow over the end of the stent. Expandable wire stents are also being used for patients with SVCO. The stent is introduced percutaneously and manipulated transvenously to the site of vena caval com-pression. Immediate relief of symptoms is usual but reocclusion will occur in 10%–20% of cases.

Other Treatments

Disease-Specific Treatments

Antibiotics
When a chest infection is contributing to breathlessness, antibiotics should be considered. The type of antibiotic will depend on the clinical setting. Neutro-

penic patients on active treatment will require broad-spectrum antibiotics to be given intravenously. Other supportive measures, including intubation and respiratory support, may be necessary in extraordinary circumstances.

In the palliative-care setting, oral antibiotics are usually satisfactory. Most exacerbations of bronchitis will respond with cavitation and foul-smelling sputum, and require anoxycillin and metronidazole or clindamycin. Atypical pneumonia should be treated with erythromycin or a tetracyclin.

Pleural Effusions

Malignant pleural effusions which become large enough to cause breathlessness should be drained. When the patient is very ill and near death, a single pleural tap removing one litre will usually be sufficient to provide relief. Usually however, a chest drain is appropriate and gradual drainage of fluid is maintained for 2–3 days. If the effusion is drained too quickly, the patient will develop chest pain and possibly unilateral pulmonary oedema. Occasionally, a pneumothorax will occur, but unless this is caused by a bronchopleural fistula, resolution will be rapid and complete.

If reaccumulation occurs or is likely, sclerosing agents may be introduced into the interpleural space. Typically, talc or tetracycline are used after the effusion is drained to dryness. A local anaesthetic is often put into the pleural space as well to minimise the inflammatory pain. If successful, the effusion will not recur or it will be confined to small pockets. Unfortunately, pleuradhesis is not always complete and significant build-up will cause further dyspnoea. The fluid will be loculated and difficult to drain. Regular diuretics, including spironolactone 100–200 mg daily, and frusemide 20 mg daily, may be helpful.

Occasionally, pleural effusions occur when ascitic fluid drains via the diaphragm into the pleural cavity. Pleuradhesis is very difficult in this situation and efforts should be directed at controlling the ascites. Rarely, free drainage of an effusion via a chest drain or open wound into a colostomy bag may be the only alternative to provide relief of dyspnoea. Surprisingly, infection is rarely a problem but the patient loses significant quantities of protein-laden fluid. A pleuro–peritoneal shunt is another alternative.

Pericardial Effusions

An unrecognised pericardial effusion with tamponade will cause rapid deterioration and death. If recognised, drainage of the effusion will produce an almost 'miraculous' recovery in many instances. A pericardial 'window' can then provide a more long-term solution if the patient is well enough to have surgery. This allows the pericardial fluid to drain into the pleural cavity. Unfortunately, some patients have extensive pericardial involvement with malignancy and the results of treatment are poor. Diuretics should be avoided when tamponade is diagnosed.

Pneumonitis

High-dose steroids are usually recommended. There is no evidence that antibiotics are helpful.

Anticoagulants

The use of anticoagulants in patients with advanced cancer is problematic. The risk of haemorrhage is increased because of the higher incidences of peptic ulceration in these patients, and because of the potential for bleeding from primary and secondary tumours. This potential is highest for vascular tumours, such as melanoma and renal cell carcinoma, as well as fungating lesions on the skin, gut or bronchial tree. The risk must be balanced against the symptoms from peripheral thromboses or emboli, and in the case of the latter, the risk of sudden death. If anticoagulants are considered, the patient must be fully informed of the risks/benefits and be involved in the decision.

In some instances, thrombosis of a major vein can be thrombolysed via a transvenous catheter. Low-dose warfarin is now used for patients with Hickman in-dwelling catheters and is being recommended for women receiving chemotherapy for breast cancer. Unfortunately, conventional doses of warfarin are often not effective clinically for patients with symptomatic thromboembolism and advanced cancer. Intermittent subcutaneous heparin injections can be more effective and can be used in the home-care setting.

Bronchodilators
Patients with lung cancer and breathlessness warrant a trial of bronchodilators, as do any other patients with a history of smoking and chronic destructive pulmonary disease. Salbutamol is given at a dose of 2.5 mg via a nebuliser at six-hourly intervals. Ipratropium, an anticholinergic agent, can also be used via a nebuliser. The dose is 0.5 mg, which can be mixed with salbutamol. Ipratropium has the potential advantage of helping to reduce secretions in patients with chronic bronchitis. Oral bronchodilators are rarely helpful and most patients have difficulty in managing inhalers. Many patients find the nebuliser masks claustrophobic. This heightens their dyspnoea. A T-piece for the mouth, or just inhalation of the vapour without a mask, will overcome this fear. Corticosteroids have a bronchodilator effect, but their use in managing dyspnoea is considered below.

Transfusion
Symptomatic anaemia (haemoglobin less that 9.0 g/l) should be treated with transfusion, unless the patient's death is imminent. Those with advanced disease tolerate fluid loads less well. This is not a reason for avoiding transfusion but the aim should be to give the minimum number of units necessary to relieve the symptoms. For patients who are transfusion-dependent, for example, those with bone-marrow failure, the response to each transfusion should be reviewed. At some point in the illness, it will be apparent that transfusions are no longer helpful.

Symptomatic Treatments

Despite the variety of anti-cancer and other specific treatments for dyspnoea, most patients will require symptomatic measures. Some measures may possibly improve exercise capacity: corticosteroids, opioids, diuretics and physiotherapy.

Corticosteroids
Steroids have a multiplicity of effects which are beneficial to breathless patients. Bronchodilatation may occur in patients with underlying asthma and chronic

bronchitis. Reduction of peritumour oedema will be useful in alleviating compression, this being the basis for using steroids in treating SVCO and upper airway obstruction. Some patients with lymphangitis will respond, suggesting some relief in the lymphatic obstruction.

The systemic effects of steroids are also helpful. Many patients will experience an improved sense of appetite and well-being for which they are greatly appreciative. Steroids have an antiemetic effect, allowing other antiemetics to be replaced if a breathless patient is also feeling nauseated. The anti-cancer effect of steroids may play a very limited role with some malignancies such as breast cancer and lymphoma.

The usual starting dose is 16 mg dexamethasone given once daily in the morning. Very breathless patients may need the dose to be administered parenterally. Higher doses can be justified if a partial effect is forthcoming, but generally the intent is to reduce the maintenance dose to the lowest possible. However, patients with a very short prognosis may be kept on the initial dose to prevent any sudden exacerbation of breathlessness. Although a therapeutic trial of one month is usually recommended for patients with chronic obstructive pulmonary disease, most cancer patients will respond within 2–3 days. If no response occurs, other options should be tried rather than allowing the patient to remain dyspnoeic.

Side-effects limit the usefulness of steroids. Fluid retention may theoretically increase breathlessness but this is unusual in practice. More worrying is the myopathy that occurs with longer-term use. The inability to get out of a chair or climb stairs can be just as disabling, even more so, than breathlessness. The timing of the introduction of steroids needs careful consideration if the prognosis is expected to be several months. The use of high-dose inhaled steroids may overcome these problems but there is no evidence supporting their use in patients with dyspnoea due to cancer.

Opioids

Following the recognition of the value of opioids in managing cancer pain, it was quickly recognised that respiratory depression was not a major clinical problem. Fortunately, this fear has been laid to rest for breathless patients as well. The careful and appropriate titration of opioids can relieve dyspnoea without causing hypoxia or hypercapnia.

The mechanisms by which opioids relieve dyspnoea are not understood. Opioids may have a sedative effect but most patients do not appreciate sedative doses being used. Patients who do use opioids to make themselves sleepy find they become tolerant to the effect and must keep increasing the dose. Rapidly escalating doses, especially at night, should serve as a warning that unresolved fear is playing an important role.

Oral morphine can increase exercise tolerance in patients with chronic obstructive pulmonary disease. Opioid receptors are found within the major airways, but it is not clear whether their function is related to bronchodilatation. Modulation of dyspneogenic signals may be taking place at spinal cord and brainstem levels.

In opioid-naive patients, the recommended starting dose of oral morphine is 2.5–5.0 mg four hourly. This can be given as immediate-release elixir or tablets. The starting dose is normally lower than for patients with pain. Patients who are already on morphine for pain will require higher doses if they become dyspnoeic as well. Some patients may only require dosing before exertion if their dyspnoea is intermittent. Doses may be repeated at 30–60 minute intervals if necessary. A full 24 hours should elapse before the background dose is increased. It takes this time to achieve steady state. Some patients can be changed to the equivalent dose of a slow-release morphine preparation, but may prefer the flexibility and availability of effect from immediate-release dosing.

The usual side-effects of nausea and vomiting should be covered with an anti-emetic. Tolerance usually occurs after a few days allowing the antiemetic to be withdrawn. Constipation is universal and laxatives must be used. The distress of constipation is worse in dyspnoeic patients. The sedative effects of morphine are also distressing. Mild drowsiness is usual and patients must be warned of this before starting. The effect is usually transient and is minimised by the low starting dose. Some patients develop an unpleasant prolongation of the expiration phase of respiration, and occasionally a Cheyne–Stokes pattern of breathing may occur, while the patient is still alert. Alternative opioids may be tried as cross-tolerance for most opioid effects is incomplete.

A traditional alternative to oral opioids is the nebulised route. Doses ranging from 5–50 mg of morphine or diamorphine have been administered by nebuliser, sometimes in combination with bronchodilators. Systemic absorption is low, suggesting a local effect in the major airways. However, a definitive study comparing nebulised morphine with placebo did not show any difference (Davis and Ahern, 1996). Meanwhile, a trial should be considered for patients who are intolerant of the central effects of morphine. The problems of using a nebuliser for breathless patients have been addressed above (see Bronchodilators, page 39).

Diuretics

Diuretics have a specific role in relieving the dyspnoea associated with heart failure. Some patients with lymphangitis may respond dramatically to diuretics. Patients with dyspnoea associated with peripheral oedema may also benefit. Some of these patients have hypoalbuminaemia which reduces renal perfusion and promotes salt/water retention. Spironolactone 100–200 mg daily, sometimes with a small dose of frusemide, will help minimise any contribution from this effect. Gentle diuresis may be necessary to help relieve the effects of peripheral oedema in severe SVCO.

Physiotherapy

Physiotherapists can provide valuable assistance in managing dyspnoea. Breathing exercises can help improve respiratory reserve. A review of daily activities can help to redirect patients' efforts into energy-efficient tasks, while avoiding the need to undertake more than one activity at a time. Formal relaxation techniques can be taught along with strategies to ease dyspnoea attacks. Aids to mobility, such as wheelchairs, can further increase patients' capabilities.

Benzodiazepines

Because anxiety is commonly associated with breathlessness, benzodiazepines are often prescribed. In general, shorter-acting examples, such as lorazepam, should be used, but chronically anxious patients may benefit from a continuous low dose of diazepam such as 2 mg 6 hourly supplemented by 5–10 mg at night.

This group of drugs rarely provides dramatic relief and many patients are treated by the residual sedative effects.

When patients are dying, the water-soluble benzodiazepine midazolam can be used as a useful adjunct to morphine. It can be mixed with morphine and delivered by continuous subcutaneous infusion of 30–60 mg per 24 hours. Single doses of 5–10 mg may be used to relieve distress within minutes.

Phenothiazines and Related Major Tranquillisers
Chlorpromazine and haloperidol have been more widely used for dyspnoea in the past. However, their use has largely been replaced by midazolam. Most patients find the sedative effect to be unpleasant if they are still alert. The antiemetic effect of these drugs should prompt their use in patients who are nauseated and breathless. Extra-pyramidal side-effects are rarely a problem.

Buspirone
The search for anxiolytics which do not cause sedation has led to the use of buspirone, a non-sedating partial serotonin agonist. The slow onset of action limits its usefulness and it must be considered early if at all. The usual starting dose is 5 mg three times daily, increasing to 15 mg at weekly intervals. Side-effects are rare. There is some evidence that buspirone increases capacity in patients with chronic obstructive pulmonary disease.

Nabilone
Nabilone is a synthetic cannabinoid that has been used as an antiemetic. It has anxiolytic and bronchodilator effects. The anticholinergic and psychotropic effects have limited its usefulness in clinical practice. However, nabilone should be considered in patients with rapidly progressive dyspnoea which is not responding to other options. Lower doses, 0.1–0.3 mg, can be given at 30 minute intervals until the dyspnoea is relieved. The total loading dose can then be repeated at 12-hourly intervals.

Local Anaesthetics
Lignocaine and bupivacaine have been nebulised for dyspnoea. Recent studies have failed to support their efficacy for this indication.

Oxygen
Several studies have shown that oxygen is superior to placebo (air) in relieving breathlessness in patients with advanced cancer. The effect is modest, reducing dyspnoea on a visual analogue scale by 20%, but occurs whether the patient has normal oxygen saturation or is hypoxic. Long-term studies are needed to confirm whether the acute effect is sustained. In practice, the impression is that oxygen therapy does not prevent progression of dyspnoea and many patients become reliant through fear of stopping rather than efficacy. Dryness of the mouth and throat and the inconvenience of nasal prongs also produce increasing problems for patients on continuous oxygen. The expense of oxygen cylinders can be ameliorated by the use of portable oxygen extraction units. The judicious use of other measures described above often obviates the need for oxygen. Few hospices in the United Kingdom use oxygen to any significant extent.

Support for the Family

Watching a breathless patient can be very distressing, especially for the family. They must be included in treatment plans if the patient is to be cared for at home. Time should be made available for the family to ask questions and share their fears. Reassurance that the patient is very unlikely to choke to death will be necessary. The family should be taught how to give immediate-release morphine, use the nebuliser and help the patient relax. These active measures will off-set the sense of helplessness. Outside support should be offered, especially if a palliative-care home-care service is available. An after-hours service will be very important. General practitioners who offer a contact telephone number rarely find that it is abused. If a hospice in-patient unit is considered, early referral will minimise delays in admission when the patient deteriorates.

Terminal Breathlessness

The usual goals of treatment for breathlessness are to maximise functional capability, relieve the distress of dyspnoea and minimise sedation. However, when severe breathlessness occurs suddenly in a patient who is dying, or when a breathless patient refuses treatment until very near the end, it is not possible to titrate therapy to relieve dyspnoea and prevent sedation. Very weak, dying patients tolerate symptoms very badly. Urgent measures will be required, with diamorphine and midazolam being given subcutaneously to maximise speed of onset of effect. For opioid-naive patients, 2.5–5 mg doses of diamorphine can be repeated at 30 minute intervals. Midazolam can be given as 5–10 mg increments at 15 minute intervals. Relatives must be warned that the patient's condition will deteriorate quickly. This is not due to the sedative effect of the drugs but to relief of the stimulant effect of the breathlessness.

Cough

Cough is another relatively common symptom. Of the patients admitted to St Christopher's Hospice, 40% cough at some time. Cough can be very distressing, particularly if the patient is very weak. Normally, cough serves a very important protective function clearing secretions from the lungs. This function should be preserved as long as possible, with treatment being aimed at the cause of the cough rather than at cough suppression. However, when a patient is dying and is too weak to clear secretions, cough should be aggressively suppressed to prevent unnecessary distress to the patient.

Causes

Cancer Related

Many of the causes of breathlessness also cause cough. Bronchial obstruction, lymphangitis carcinomatosa, pleural effusions and tracheal narrowing can all be associated with a dry irritating cough. Vocal cord paralysis can cause cough as well as a hoarse voice. Distal accumulation of secretions will exacerbate cough. Intra-alveolar cancer can produce copious quantities of a surfactant-like material and hence a very productive cough. Lung metastases do not usually cause cough unless bronchial obstruction occurs.

Squamous-cell lung cancers frequently undergo necrosis. Secondary infection can result in a foul-smelling productive cough typical of a lung abscess. Cancers which cause difficulty in swallowing, for example, head and neck cancer, may lead to aspiration and infection. Nocturnal cough can result from gastric reflux with spill-over of acid into the trachea. This occurs in patients who have had gastro-oesophageal surgery, or who have raised intra-abdominal pressure from gross ascites, for example.

Treatment Related

Pneumonitis from radiotherapy or chemotherapy agents can produce a dry cough which is more distressing than breathlessness. Immune suppressed patients on chemotherapy are at risk of developing chest infections with cough.

Other Conditions

The association between chronic obstructive pulmonary disease and asthma with lung cancer has been noted. Both of these diseases cause chronic cough which will be made worse by acute bronchitis. Pneumonias may occur in cancer patients who are not on treatment.

Treatments

Oncological

Radiotherapy is effective for cough from endobronchial obstruction but has no value in treating lymphangitis and other disseminated intrapulmonary causes. Chemotherapy may work if the disease is responsive. Other treatments for endobronchial lesions such as stenting can also be useful.

Disease Specific

These include:

(a) *Antibiotics*. A productive cough from a chest infection is an indication for appropriate antibiotic therapy. However, any decision to start antibiotics should be reviewed if the patient is dying.
(b) *Pleural effusions*. Malignant pleural effusions should be drained, as described above.
(c) *Pneumonitis*. High-dose steroids are recommended but may not relieve the cough.
(d) *Bronchodilators*. These, especially ipratropium, can minimise sputum production and improve patients' ability to clear sputum.

Symptomatic Treatments

Patients who are dying require symptomatic treatments for cough. Options include:

(a) *Opioids*. These reduce the perception of cough. Frequently, patients are already on morphine for cancer pain but the dose can be increased if necessary for cough. Respiratory depression will not happen.
(b) *Cough linctus*. There are many examples of cough linctus available, some of which contain small doses of opioid. It is the syrup base which probably helps to relieve cough.
(c) *Diuretics*. These may relieve cough associated with lymphangitis.
(d) *Local anaesthetics*. Lignocaine and bupivacaine can be nebulised for persistent dry unproductive cough. They are more effective for this indication than for treating dyspnoea.
(e) *Anticholinergics*. These drugs can reduce the secretions associated with productive cough. Hyoscine hydrobromide (scopolamine) is often given by subcutaneous injection when patients are dying, usually at a dose of 0.2–0.4 mg four hourly. Hyoscine transdermal patches are effective and less sedating for patients who are not actually dying. Alternatively, glycopyrronium is also less sedating and can be given by injection (0.1–0.2 mg four hourly or by continuous infusion). Mention has already been made of ipratropium; atropine can also be given by nebuliser.
(f) *Sedatives*. Sometimes, the only way to relieve distressing cough in a dying patient is to use sedatives. Hyoscine injections will have this effect but medications such as midazolam (5–10 mg) may be needed.

Haemoptysis

Introduction

Haemoptysis, which is the coughing up of blood, is much less common than the other two major respiratory symptoms. When it occurs, there is usually small streaks of blood associated with sputum or small quantities of fresh blood, less than one teaspoonful. Occasionally, however, the bleeding may be persistent. If haemoptysis is very significant such as occurs with erosion of a major bronchial artery, the patient will exsanguinate within minutes. It is the fear of this possibility that worries patients who have minimal haemoptysis. Fortunately, death from haemoptysis is rare but the symptom should be considered as important no matter how insignificant the quantity of blood seems.

Causes of Haemoptysis

Cancer Related

Lung cancers are far and away the commonest malignant causes of haemoptysis. Primary bronchial lesions may bleed from an ulcerated necrotic surface or may erode into a bronchial artery. Haemoptysis from lung metastases is rare because they tend to remain intrapulmonary. Any bleeding disorder or infection associated with an intrabronchial lesion will increase the likelihood and the severity of haemoptysis.

Treatment Related

Haemoptysis following anti-cancer treatments is extremely rare. Severe thrombocytopenia associated with chemotherapy agents is a potential cause if there is a predisposing site that is bleeding. Spontaneous bleeding from an extremely low platelet count normally arises from the gums, gastrointestinal tract, or occasionally into the brain.

Other Conditions

It is unwise to attribute haemoptysis to acute bronchitis or other chest infection in patients with lung cancer and pre-existing chronic obstructive pulmonary disease unless the cancer is excluded as the cause.

Pulmonary embolism associated with infarction is a possibility but can be difficult to prove. It should be suspected in patients who do not have known lung cancer or lung metastases. Pulmonary angiography is the 'gold standard' test but carries some risk, particularly if the patient is otherwise very unwell. Ventilation/perfusion lung scans are less risky but also more inaccurate if other causes of lung disease are present.

Oncological Treatments

Radiotherapy is the standard treatment for cancer-related haemoptysis. External beam therapy is usually given but brachytherapy is available in some centres. The tendency is to give one or two doses if the patient has a poor prognosis. It is even possible to give a single fraction if the patient has already had maximal doses to treat the primary lesion if the prognosis is poor and long-term effects are not likely. Laser and cryotherapy have been used to control haemorrhage. Surgery is rarely an option but may be considered if asphyxiation is a risk and the patient's general condition is otherwise very good.

Other Treatments

Disease Specific

Antibiotics
Antibiotics can be used if there is evidence that a chest infection is contributing to haemoptysis, but should not be considered as a first or only choice. They are likely to help if there is cavitation and anaerobic infection.

Anticoagulants
The risks of anticoagulating patients with advanced cancer have already been outlined. However, if a patient is otherwise well but has a proven pulmonary embolism, the risk of sudden death from further embolus must be assessed. A decision to anticogulate will be difficult and should involve advice from specialists as well as informed discussion with the patient.

Transfusion
Symptomatic anaemia rarely arises from haemoptysis. Other blood products, such as platelets and fresh-frozen plasma, may be required to correct coagulopathies.

Symptomatic

Most instances of haemoptysis will be fleeting and resolve spontaneously. Keeping the patient calm and advising bed rest are helpful general measures if the haemoptysis is more persistent.

Antifibrinolytics
There are several antifibrinolytic agents such as tranexamic acid which could theoretically control haemoptysis when active treatments have failed or are not appropriate. They are widely used but there is no evidence that they are of any benefit, except perhaps to the prescriber. There is the risk of stroke and myocardial infarction with this group of drugs.

Opioids

If a patient has a large haemoptysis, a stat injection of morphine or diamorphine will help to ease the fear and lower the blood pressure.

Benzodiazepines

When haemoptysis is a terminal event, the addition of a rapid acting benzo-diazepene such as midazolam (5–20 mg) to the morphine will render the patient unaware of what is happening.

Support for the Family

When a patient dies of haemoptysis, the family will need a lot of support. The death will have occurred unexpectedly. The trauma of the timing will be compounded if the family witnessed the death. Many weeks or months of counselling will be necessary if they were not prepared for the death or were not supported at the time that the patient was dying. If the possibility of a major haemoptysis is known and further active treatment is not possible, the patient need not be automatically admitted to an institution. With proper community backup, some families are able to cope with the possibility.

4 – Gastrointestinal Symptoms in Oncology

by Nigel Sykes and Mary Baines

Introduction

Gastrointestinal symptoms are commonly associated with advanced cancer. Some of these symptoms are easily recognised, for example, dysphagia associated with oesophageal cancer and intestinal obstruction associated with inoperable bowel cancer. However, many patients suffer unnecessarily from symptoms such as constipation and nausea, which are more common but less obvious. This chapter reviews the management of dysphagia, constipation, diarrhoea, nausea and vomiting, and intestinal obstruction.

Dysphagia

Introduction

In a general population of patients with advanced cancer the prevalence of dysphagia is about 12%. The majority of cases are due to either oesophageal tumours or high gastric tumours, but 80% of those with head and neck cancer also have dysphagia.

Causes

Most cases of dysphagia associated with malignancy are due to obstruction to the passage of food by tumour masses within the oesophagus, at the cardia or compressing the oesophagus from outside. However, splinting or anatomical distortion of the pharynx as a result of oro-pharyngeal cancer or the ensuing surgery and radiotherapy may also contribute. Perineural spread of pharyngeal cancers can occur, disrupting co-ordination of oesophageal peristalsis (Carter et al., 1982).

Orofacial or neck pain can inhibit swallowing, and a cause of uncomfortable swallowing which should not be overlooked is candidal infection. This may be present in the oesophagus even in the absence of oral thrush.

Of cancer patients undergoing palliation, 30% who complain of dysphagia have no objective evidence of swallowing difficulty (Sykes et al., 1988). This group predominantly has tumours distant from the upper digestive tract, and their symptom appears to be due to poor appetite or anxiety.

Management

The patient's swallowing should be observed, noting the consistency of food that can be swallowed and whether swallowing is accompanied by pain or cough. Candidal infection characteristically gives pain on swallowing hot liquids, and cough suggests the presence of an oesophago-tracheal fistula.

Any distressing symptom will exacerbate dysphagia through anxiety or reduction of appetite, so the management of swallowing problems requires good general symptom control and a supportive environment. This is especially evident for those with no known tumour deposits around the upper gastrointestinal tract, whose complaint of dysphagia often disappears when they gain an improved sense of comfort and security.

Head and neck cancer patients are likely to have an impaired ability to form or transfer food boluses, and to initiate swallowing. A speech therapy assessment can be invaluable in providing aids to eating and drinking, and in teaching manoeuvres to circumvent the functional impairment.

Overall, about 60% of patients with malignant dysphagia can be helped by conservative treatment. This depends principally on careful attention to provision of food that the individual likes, of the consistency they can manage, presented as attractively as possible. Liquid food supplements are valuable, but a food blender can render most conventional meals into an appropriate consistency. The result will be more appetising if attention is paid to garnishing. People whose eating is slow need the means for hot food to be kept at the right temperature throughout the meal. Size of portions should reflect the patient's appetite and be reflected in the size of the plate on which they are served.

These methods enable the most to be made of an impaired swallowing ability and also encourage appetite. Appetite stimulation by steroids or megestrol acetate is valuable as long as it does not produce hunger in excess of the capacity to swallow. By reduction of peritumour oedema, steroids may directly improve dysphagia, especially, it appears, when it is associated with the perineural spread of cancer.

Specific Treatments

For many patients with advanced disease referred for palliation, only conservative treatment is available for dysphagia. However, for patients fit enough, various methods exist to reduce tumour narrowing of the oesophageal lumen.

Surgery may be the best palliation of oesophageal cancer but is possible for only about 40%. Chemotherapy may occasionally be relevant for external compression caused by mediastinal nodal spread from chemosensitive disease elsewhere.

Oesophageal dilatation can improve swallowing in 92% of cases and in practised hands has a perforation rate of under 0.01% (Heit et al., 1978). Its benefits are temporary, however, unless it is followed by intubation, and this is probably the best procedure for relieving dysphagia in patients with a short prognosis for whom repeated hospital visits are unacceptable. It is also widely available.

Endoscopic intubation of the oesophagus using, for instance, an Atkinson tube, alleviates dysphagia in 90%–100% of patients initially and in 85%–90% for the rest of their lives. It is appropriate for external compression and for the closure of tracheo-oesophageal fistulae. The mortality of the procedure is 3%–16%, with perforation and tube displacement as major complications, and reflux and tube blockage more minor, but potentially distressing, ones.

The quality of swallowing provided by oesophageal tubes is usually far from normal: 10%–15% of patients can eat a virtually normal diet if permitted to do so, 50%–60% a semi-solid diet and the rest liquids only. Nd:YAG laser removal of oesophageal tumour improves swallowing in a similar proportion of patients, but at least 30% can swallow a normal diet (Loizou et al., 1992). Complications may be less than with intubation but repeated treatments are necessary, often at intervals of four weeks or so, resulting in an increased total time in hospital even though a proportion of cases can be treated on an out-patient basis. Laser equipment is expensive, with consequent restriction in its availability, but the technique may provide better results than intubation in relatively well patients in whom it can be repeated if beneficial.

External-beam radiotherapy for oesophageal cancer has not been shown to offer efficient palliation of dysphagia. However, a single fraction of intra-cavitary irradiation using after-loaded caesium or iridium sources in an endoscopically placed application tube has been claimed to give good relief of dysphagia in 65% of cases with a median duration of 14 weeks (Rowland and Pagliero, 1985). The incidence of oesophagitis is unclear, as is any advantage over laser therapy.

Two cheaper alternatives to either laser or irradiation are electro-coagulation and ethanol-induced tumour necrosis. The former is applicable to encircling lesions of the oesophagus and produces results of the same quality and duration as those of laser treatment (Jensen et al., 1988). The latter is based on the technique of injection of sclerosant solutions into oesophageal varices. Again, the results are claimed to be comparable with those of laser treatment but at a fraction of the cost.

Further comparative work is needed for any judgement to be made regarding the relative merits of the various methods of palliation for dysphagia caused by oesophageal tumour. The treatment an individual receives will be determined by local availability as much as by merit (Table 4.1).

Table 4.1 Methods of palliation of malignant dysphagia

Conservative	Specific
Good general symptom control	Oesophageal dilatation
Oral hygiene	Oesophageal intubation
Food of correct type and consistency	Nd:YAG laser
Appetite stimulation	Intracavitary radiotherapy
Steroids	Electrocoagulation
	Ethanol-induced tumour necrosis

Constipation

Introduction

The normal range of bowel function is very wide: 99% of British people defaecate between three times a day and three times a week. Hence, rather than seeking objective criteria of constipation, it is better to accept the condition as a subjective symptom and define it as difficulty and discomfort in defaecation. Current indices of bowel function, such as frequency, are then compared with the individual's own norms.

About 10% of a normal population consider themselves constipated and, despite many already receiving laxatives, around 50% of patients with advanced cancer do so.

Causes

Drugs, especially opioid analgesics, are frequently blamed for constipation in cancer patients. However, 63% of such patients who do not take opioids still require laxatives. This suggests a strong underlying constipating effect of debility, probably mediated through reduced food and fluid intake and restricted physical activity. Nevertheless, strong opioid analgesia is the largest single identifiable constipating factor in this patient group: 87% of those on oral morphine or diamorphine require laxatives. No significant tolerance to this effect appears to develop, but lower morphine doses are proportionately more constipating than higher ones.

Management

The initial step is to discover the present bowel habit and that accepted as normal, and to make a rectal and abdominal examination in order to exclude faecal impaction and intestinal obstruction. It is not always easy to distinguish obstruction from severe constipation, abdominal radiology occasionally being necessary.

Good general symptom control maximises the ability to eat and to mobilise, which will reduce the tendency to constipation. Additional dietary fibre has to be provided carefully, as it is poorly tolerated by ill patients and is largely ineffective in marked constipation; Mumford (1986) found that a 50% increase in stool frequency of patients in a radiotherapy unit would require a 450% increase in their fibre intake.

The majority of cancer patients requiring palliation are likely to need laxatives. These should be started in anticipation of constipating drugs, whether opioids, antidepressants or vincristine, and the dose individually titrated against the response and the patient's satisfaction.

Despite extensive use of oral laxatives, about 40% of patients continue to be given suppositories or enemas or both. Not surprisingly, a majority of people prefer oral to rectal treatment and so this route of treatment must be made as effective as possible.

Laxatives are conventionally, if inaccurately, divided into drugs that predominantly soften stool and those that predominantly stimulate colonic peristalsis (Table 4.2). The combination of a stimulant and a softener is effective at a lower dose than that of a softener alone and with less risk of colic than a stimulant alone. Use of a softener, such as lactulose, by itself is unlikely to be adequate for most patients receiving opioids.

Laxatives should be titrated in dose in the same way as analgesics. There is no correct dose, except that which controls the individual's constipation to their satisfaction. Colic implies that too little softening agent is present relative to the stimulant; an intolerable volume of laxative indicates a change to a more effective agent.

Few comparative studies are available to guide the choice of laxatives. The commonly used combination of lactulose with senna is more potent than normal strength codanthramer (see Table 4.2) but probably less than the higher strength. Per unit volume, codanthrusate suspension falls between the two codanthramer preparations in potency. Magnesium hydroxide emulsion with liquid paraffin may be used simply as a softener with senna, but potentially has stimulant actions as well and can substitute for the senna/lactulose combination at a higher dose but still at lower cost. Anecdotally, bisacodyl and sodium picosulphate are more potent stimulants than senna. Saline laxatives, such as magnesium sulphate, may still be useful for resistant constipation.

The only primarily stimulant rectal laxative preparation is the suppository of bisacodyl. Other commonly used rectal agents, such as glycerine suppositories, oil enemas and the various proprietary varieties of phosphate enemas and mini-enemas, mainly soften stool. The reflex response to rectal distension and the saline component of some preparations probably produce colonic contraction as well. Both enemas and suppositories elicit defaecation on over 80% of occasions, with a median latency of about 30 min for enemas and 60 min for suppositories.

An approach to the management of constipation, and the use of laxatives, is suggested in Table 4.3.

Table 4.2   Commonly used laxatives

Predominantly softening			
Mode of action	Examples	Usual dose range	Comment
Osmotic agents: Retain water in gut lumen	Lactulose	15–40 ml bd – tds	Active principally in the small bowel. Latency of action 1–2 days.
	Magnesium hydroxide Magnesium sulphate	2–4 g daily	Act throughout the bowel and may have pronounced purgative effect, possibly partly as a result of direct peristaltic stimulation. Latency of action 1–6 hours (dose dependent).
Surfactant agents: Increase water penetration of the stool	Docusate sodium Poloxamer (only available in combination with danthron)	Docusate 60–300 mg bd	Probably not very effective when used alone. Latency of action 1–3 days.
Lubricant agents:	Liquid paraffin Glycerine (as suppositories) Arachis oil Olive oil (as enemas)		Paraffin is best used only in a 25% emulsion with magnesium hydroxide (Mil-Par)

Predominantly stimulant			
Direct stimulation of myenteric nerves to induce peristalsis. Reduce absorption of water from gut.	Senna Danthron	7.5–30 mg bd 50–450 mg bd	Anthraquinone family. Danthron available only in combination with docusate or poloxamer – stains urine red/brown Latency of action 6–12 h.
	Bisacodyl Sodium picosulphate	10–20 mg bd 5–20 mg bd	Polyphenolic family. Latency of action 6–12 h.

Combination stimulant/softener preparations			
Codanthramer standard	Danthron 25 mg with Poloxamer 200 mg per 5 ml or capsule		Suspension or capsule
Codanthramer forte	Danthron 75 mg with Poloxamer 1 g per 5 ml or 2 capsules		Suspension or capsule
Codanthrusate	Danthron 50 mg with Docusate 60 mg per 5 ml or capsule		Capsule or suspension
Emulsion magnesium hydroxide and liquid paraffin (3:1 ratio)			Liquid only

Table 4.3   Management of constipation

1. Take adequate prophylactic measures:

   - Maintain good general symptom control
   - Encourage activity
   - Maintain adequate oral fluid intake
   - Maximise the fibre content of the diet
   - Anticipate constipating effects of drugs, altering treatment or starting a laxative prophylactically
   - Ensure privacy and dignity

2. Despite prophylaxis, most patients with advanced cancer will reqire laxatives. There is no single correct way of selecting and using laxatives, but here is a summary of one rational approach:

   - *Exclude intestinal obstruction by examination, and, if necessary, radiography.* If doubt remains, use only laxatives with a predominantly softening action, e.g. lactulose or sodium docusate, in order to avoid causing colic. Do not use bulking agents.
   - *If the rectum is impacted with hard faeces:* Spontaneous evacuation is unlikely to be possible without local measures to soften the faecal mass, e.g. glycerine suppositories, olive or arachis oil enema. It still may be necessary to perform a manual rectal evacuation, for which sedation or additional analgesia is often required.
   - *If the rectum is loaded with soft faeces:* A predominantly peristalsis-stimulating laxative, e.g. senna, may be effective alone. If there is rectal discomfort, a mini-enema may assist the initial defaecation. Frequent review is essential, as there is a likelihood that a stool-softening laxative will be required later as well, given either separately, e.g. lactulose, or in a combination preparation, e.g. codanthrusate, codanthramer.
   - *If there is little or no stool in the rectum:* A peristalsis-stimulating laxative is the drug of choice, e.g. senna, but the stools are likely to be hard and it is a reasonable policy to use a stool-softening laxative in addition, e.g. lactulose, or a combination preparation, e.g. codanthrusate, codanthramer.

Diarrhoea

Introduction

Diarrhoea occurs in 7%–10% of people with advanced cancer and so is a much smaller problem than constipation. Although defined as the frequent passage of loose stools, patients may also use diarrhoea to refer to a single loose stool, frequent normal stools or faecal incontinence.

Causes

The most common cause of diarrhoea in this patient group is an overdose of laxatives, generally occurring during dose titration to overcome existing constipation. The diarrhoea settles with a 24–48 h break from laxatives, after which they should be restarted at a lower dose in order to avoid a recurrence.

Among other common drugs, antibiotics and antacids frequently cause diarrhoea and non-steroidal anti-inflammatory drugs do so occasionally.

Sorbitol, included in various elixirs, can be a covert source of bowel disturbance.

Faecal impaction causes leakage of fluid stool past the faecal mass to give spurious diarrhoea. In an elderly population of hospital patients, faecal impaction has been reported to produce 55% of cases of diarrhoea (Kinnunen et al., 1989). Partial intestinal obstruction can produce either diarrhoea or alternating diarrhoea and constipation. Radiation directed to the abdomen or pelvis is prone to cause diarrhoea beginning in the second or third week of therapy.

Significant causes of diarrhoea in patients with advanced cancer are listed in Table 4.4.

Table 4.4   Causes of diarrhoea in advanced cancer

1. Drugs:
   - Laxatives
   - Antacids
   - Antibiotics
   - Chemotherapy agents, especially 5-fluorouracil
   - NSAIDs, especially mefenamic acid, diclofenac, indomethacin
   - Iron preparations
   - Disaccharide-containing elixirs

2. Radiation

3. Obstruction:
   - Malignant
   - Faecal impaction

4. Malabsorption:
   - Pancreatic carcinoma
   - Gastrectomy
   - Ileal resection
   - Colectomy

5. Tumours:
   - Colonic or rectal carcinoma
   - Pancreatic islet cell tumours
   - Carcinoid tumours

6. Concurrent disease:
   - Diabetes mellitus
   - Gastrointestinal infection

7. Diet

Management

A history which includes the frequency of defaecation, the type of stool and the time course of the problem often suggests the diagnosis. Profuse watery stools imply reduced colonic fluid absorption, usually due to intestinal infection. Pale, fatty, offensive stools indicate steatorrhoea caused by pancreatic or small bowel insufficiency. Diarrhoea occurring only once or twice a day may in fact be anal incontinence, while an onset after a period of constipation, often with little warning of defaecation, suggests impaction.

Intestinal obstruction and faecal impaction are usually detected on abdominal or rectal examination. Stool cultures are not usually worthwhile without a history of recent warm climate travel, HIV infection or blood in the faeces, as most infective diarrhoea will clear within the time taken to diagnose it.

Diarrhoea seen in oncology patients without HIV infection is rarely severe enough to cause dehydration, and oral fluids, possibly including appropriately formulated electrolyte solutions, are generally sufficient to replace losses.

Specific Treatments

Specific treatments are available for certain types of diarrhoea. Pancreatin, a combination of lipase, amylase and protease, replaces pancreatic enzyme deficiency. The dose required must be individually determined and may be reduced if an H_2 antagonist is also given.

Aspirin, prednisolone enemas and the rather unpalatable cholestyramine are all claimed to help radiation-induced diarrhoea.

Symptomatic Treatments

Although various absorbent (e.g. methyl cellulose) and adsorbent (e.g. kaolin) agents exist, the principal symptomatic treatments of diarrhoea are opioids. Codeine (10–60 mg four hourly) is the cheapest antidiarrhoeal drug but has marked systemic effects. Diphenoxylate (up to 20 mg per day) is more potent and has fewer systemic effects but the atropine which is combined with it to limit abuse may cause adverse effects. The drug of choice is loperamide (up to 16 mg per day), which is minimally absorbed and so has very few general opioid effects.

Nausea and Vomiting

Introduction

Nausea, vomiting and retching are common and distressing complaints. Various surveys have put the prevalence of one or more of these at between 40% and 60% of patients with advanced cancer.

Pathophysiology

An understanding of the emetic process and the common neurotransmitters involved is helpful in assessing and treating the patient who is vomiting. Antiemetic drugs are effective at different receptor sites and are therefore useful in treating different causes of vomiting. The emetic centre (or possibly a chain of effector nuclei) can be stimulated in the following ways:

- From the chemoreceptor trigger zone (CTZ), where dopamine and serotonin (5-HT) receptors are concentrated.
- From vagal and sympathetic afferents from the gastrointestinal tract.
- From the vestibular centre. This, like the emetic centre, contains both histamine and muscarinic cholinergic receptors.
- From raised intracranial pressure.
- From psychological causes, especially anxiety.

Causes

The principal causes of nausea and vomiting in advanced malignancy are given in Table 4.5.

Table 4.5   Common causes of vomiting in the patient with advanced cancer

Chemical causes:
- Drugs, especially opioids and chemotherapy
- Uraemia
- Hypercalcaemia
- Infection

Gastric causes:
- Gastritis or ulceration
- Gashic stasis due to drugs, especially opioids
- External pressure causing 'squashed stomach syndrome'
- Carcinoma of stomach
- Gastroduodenal obstruction

Intestinal obstruction
Abdominal or pelvic radiotherapy
Constipation
Raised intracranial pressure
Vestibular disturbance
Cough-induced
Anxiety

Management

The causes of vomiting in the patient with advanced cancer can usually be determined from a careful history and clinical examination. Note should also be taken of the volume, content and timing of vomits. A biochemical profile may be needed but other investigations are often inappropriate.

Nausea can be treated with oral medication, but alternative routes are needed for the patient with severe vomiting. An antiemetic injection is suitable to control a single episode of vomiting but, with a persistent problem, it is preferable to give drugs by subcutaneous infusion using a syringe driver or similar device. Antiemetics (in suppository or tablet form) can also be given rectally.

In a few patients, the specific cause of vomiting can be identified and treated successfully (Table 4.6). However, the majority of patients have irreversible and multiple causes of vomiting; they will require treatment with antiemetics and other measures.

Table 4.6   Reversible causes of vomiting

Cause of vomiting	Treatment
Hypercalcaemia	Rehydration and bisphosphonates
Infection	Antibiotics
Raised intracranial pressure	Dexamethasone
Gastric irritation or ulceration	Stop NSAID. Give H_2 antagonist or misoprostol
Constipation	Rectal measures and laxatives
Anxiety	Explanation and reassurance
	Anxiolytic drugs

There are a large number of antiemetic drugs, effective at different sites in the emetic cycle and therefore of use in different causes of vomiting. The drugs are shown in Table 4.7; the following is the usual approach to the management of vomiting from different causes:

- Opioid-induced vomiting. About 30% of patients starting morphine feel nauseated during the first week of treatment. Either metoclopramide or haloperidol should be given prophylactically to cover this period.
- Cytotoxic chemotherapy. Ondansetron is the drug of choice, sometimes given with dexamethasone. High dose metoclopramide and dexamethasone is a less-effective but less-expensive alternative. Lorazepam reduces anticipatory nausea and vomiting.
- Renal failure. Haloperidol is usually effective, methotrimeprazine is sometimes required for intractable vomiting.
- Squashed stomach syndrome. This is usually due to hepatomegaly and is treated with metoclopramide or domperidone.
- Gastroduodenal obstruction. Metoclopramide may be effective if the obstruction is partial. Dexamethasone can shrink inflammatory oedema around an obstructive lesion. Octreotide may reduce the volume of vomit, otherwise nasogastric suction will be required.
- Intestinal obstruction.
- Raised intracranial pressure. If dexamethasone is contraindicated or ineffective, cyclizine is the antiemetic of choice.
- Vestibular disturbance. Both hyoscine hydrobromide and cyclizine are used.

Intestinal Obstruction

Introduction

Intestinal obstruction is caused by an occlusion to the lumen or a lack of normal propulsion which prevents or delays intestinal contents from passing along the gastrointestinal tract. Obstruction occurs in about 3% of patients with advanced cancer receiving hospice treatment (Baines, 1993) but the incidence in patients with advanced ovarian cancer is much higher, up to 40% (Beattie et al., 1989).

Table 4.7 Antiemetic drugs

Antiemetic	Dose 24/h	Main site of action
Phenothiazines		
Prochlorperazine	15–60 mg	Block dopamine receptors at CTZ
Methotrimeprazine	75–200 mg	
Butyrophenones		
Haloperidol	1.5–15 mg	Block dopamine receptors at CTZ
Antihistamines		
Cyclizine	150 mg	Vestibular and emetic centres
Anticholinergics		
Hyoscine hydrobromide	1.6–2.4 mg	Vestibular and emetic. Reduce gastrointestinal
Hyoscine butylbromide	60–300 mg	secretions and motility
Gastrokinetic		
Metoclopramide	30–80 mg	Increase peristalsis in upper gut, also dopamine
Domperidone	30–80 mg	antagonists
5-HT₃ receptor antagonists		
Ondansetron	8–16 mg	Block serotonin receptors at CTZ and in gut
Corticosteroids		
Dexamethasone	8–20 mg	Reduce inflammatory oedema. Also central effect
Somatostatin analogues		
Octreotide	0.3–0.6 mg	Reduce gastrointestinal secretions and motility

Causes

Obstruction can be caused by a mechanical occlusion due to intraluminal or intramural tumour, or to extrinsic compression from adhesions or tumour masses. Motility disorders can cause a functional obstruction (pseudo-obstruction); they are due to malignant involvement of bowel muscle, mesentery or coeliac plexus. Frequently, both mechanical and functional obstructions are present and occur at several sites in the small and/or large intestine.

Intestinal obstruction is usually caused by primary tumours of the ovary or large bowel. Gastroduodenal obstruction is much less common and is a complication of pancreatic or stomach cancer.

Clinical Features

The symptoms and signs of intestinal obstruction when it occurs at different levels in the gastrointestinal tract, are well known, and are not given here. However, what has been less well recognised is the frequent intermittent nature of obstructive symptoms. Patients are often admitted with severe vomiting and colic with no bowel action for many days. Yet the symptoms may settle spontaneously, if temporarily.

Surgical colleagues often make the distinction between complete and partial (subacute) obstruction. But this diagnosis may not be sustained and the patient who was thought to be totally obstructed (with no bowel action and minimal or no flatus) may, after some weeks, spontaneously pass a stool.

Surgery

Surgical treatment, aimed at restoring the continuity of the bowel lumen, should be considered for every patient with advanced cancer who develops intestinal obstruction. A proportion will have a non-malignant cause or an unrelated second primary tumour. The knowledge that pharmacological treatment is an effective option must not prevent a patient from receiving palliative surgery which can offer some individuals a long and symptom-free period.

However, it needs to be recognised that palliative surgery in patients with obstruction from metastatic cancer has a high operative mortality and a median survival of a few months. There is a high incidence of enterocutaneous fistulae. These usually occur in the laparotomy scar, making it difficult to fit the usual appliances, and thus greatly reduce the patient's quality of life.

These statistics indicate that patients should be selected more carefully for surgery. The options for pharmacological treatment to relieve symptoms or a venting gastrostomy may make it easier for surgical colleagues to decide against palliative surgery for some patients, knowing that these methods will prevent a distressing death from obstruction.

Gastrointestinal Intubation

The insertion of a nasogastric tube is almost routinely done when an obstructed patient, with advanced cancer, is admitted to hospital. However, a review of the surgical literature shows that, in these patients, the sustained response to such treatment is very poor, being only 0–2%. Conservative treatment should therefore be reserved for those patients who are being considered for palliative surgery while investigations are performed and the patient's wishes elucidated. If appropriate, surgery should be undertaken as soon as possible. There is no value in repeated hospital admissions with intubation and intravenous fluids in the patient with advanced cancer in the hope that this treatment will resolve the obstruction. In the majority of cases, obstructive symptoms can be controlled pharmacologically without intubation, but a small group, mainly with gastroduodenal or jejunal obstruction, require prolonged intubation or, possibly, a venting gastrostomy.

Venting Gastrostomy

A venting gastrostomy or jejunostomy can be used to relieve intractable nausea and vomiting in patients with inoperable intestinal obstruction. It is both more effective and more acceptable than prolonged nasogastric drainage. In most series, patients treated in this way were placed on a liquid diet, the gastrostomy tube being clamped at meals and for as long afterwards as could be tolerated. Good relief of nausea and vomiting were obtained and, in some, the gastrostomy output was reduced, presumably due to a remission of the obstruction (Malone et al., 1986; Gemio et al., 1986; Ashby et al., 1991).

Unfortunately, most authors describe the use of a venting gastrostomy as the primary treatment for inoperable bowel obstruction without first considering pharmacological treatment. It is probable that some patients could have been managed with medication, without recourse to surgery and tubes which inevitably add to the distress of terminal illness. Further studies are needed to define 'The small subgroup of patients who do not respond adequately to pharmacological measures and require some form of decompression or venting procedure' (Ashby et al., 1991).

Pharmacological Treatment

Drugs have been used for a number of years to relieve symptoms and the regimens have gradually evolved. Continuous subcutaneous infusion using a portable syringe driver or similar pump is the preferred route of drug administration. A combination of drugs can be given and the syringe driver is ideal for use in the home as it can be loaded every 24 hours by the visiting nurse (Johnson and Patterson, 1992). Other routes are less effective and are now rarely used except in situations where a syringe driver is unobtainable.

The main symptoms and their treatment are shown in Table 4.8. In practice, the symptoms of colic, continuous abdominal pain and vomiting occur together, and a typical prescription when treatment is started would be

diamorphine (or morphine) 30 mg
hyoscine butylbromide 60 mg
haloperidol 5 mg

given over 24 hours, by subcutaneous infusion, using a syringe driver.

If continuous pain or colic are not controlled, the dose of opioid or antispasmodic should be increased, If vomiting remains a problem, the dose of haloperidol can be increased or a change made to another antiemetic or octreotide.

The anti-inflammatory effect of corticosteroids causes reduction of peritumour inflammatory oedema. For this reason steroids have been used in some centres in the management of obstructed patients, with the expectation that they will cause an opening up of the obstruction and consequent symptom relief. There have been reports of small groups of patients who have benefited, but no clinical trials have been conducted. With the intermittent nature of early obstructive symptoms, it is difficult to know if the improvement is due to the steroid treatment.

Table 4.8   Drugs used to relieve symptoms in intestinal obstruction

Symptom	Drug	Dose/24 hours (by sub-cutaneous infusion)	Comment
Intestinal colic	Diamorphine (or morphine)	As required	Usually an antispasmodic is also used
	Hyoscine butyl-bromide	60–300 mg	Not sedating
Continuous abdominal pain	Diarmorphine (or morphine)	As required	–
Nausea and vomiting	Haloperidol	5–15 mg	Antiemetic of choice
	Cyclizine	100–200 mg	May crystallise in syringe driver
	Hyoscinem butyl-bromide	60–300 mg	Reduces gastrointestinal secretions
	Octreotide*	0.3–0.6 mg	Reduces gastrointestinal secretions
	Methotri-meprazine	50–150 mg	Very effective antiemetic. Sedating
Diarrhoea (from subacute obstruction or faecal fistula)	Codeine	60–240 mg (orally)	–
	Loperamide	6–16 mg (orally)	–
	Octreotide	0.3–0.6 mg	–

*Mercadante et al. (1993) and Riley and Fallon (1994)

Results of Pharmacological Treatment

Studies have shown that the control of continuous abdominal pain is very good, with about 90% of patients becoming pain free. Colic is harder to control and about a third continue to have mild colic. The management of nausea and vomiting is more difficult and the majority of patients continue to vomit about once a day, but experience little nausea (Baines et al., 1985; Ventafridda et al., 1990).

With good or moderate control of nausea and vomiting, patients can eat and drink as they choose. The majority favour small, low-residue and mainly fluid meals which are mostly absorbed in the proximal part of the gastrointestinal tract. With adequate oral fluids, thirst is rarely a problem and a dry mouth is treated with local measures, such as crushed ice to suck. There remains a small group of patients, mainly with gastroduodenal or jejunal obstruction, who continue to vomit profusely, in spite of medication. These may benefit from the insertion of a nasogastric tube or venting gastrostomy. Fluids can be given, if needed, by intravenous infusion or by hypodermoclysis (subcutaneous fluids). This is well tolerated and can be administered in the home by nursing staff (Fainsinger et al., 1994).

5 – Management of Other Symptoms

Introduction

This chapter covers some of the other symptoms experienced by cancer patients. The symptoms selected for this chapter occur frequently or can be very distressing Weight loss, poor appetite and weakness occur in almost all patients. Confusion and terminal restlessness are less common but no less distressing when they do occur. Hypercalcaemia and hyponatraemia are metabolic complications of cancer which cause multiple symptoms, but they are considered in the section on confusion (page 71). Mouth and skin problems can be troublesome. Convulsions are associated with brain tumours and require careful management.

Weight Loss and Poor Appetite

Cancer is associated with weight loss (cachexia) and poor appetite (anorexia) in half of the patients presenting for treatment, increasing to over 75% of patients who are terminally ill. Along with the prospect of a painful agonising death, the gaunt wasted appearance of patients with advanced cancer has contributed to the fear of cancer in the minds of the public. The distress of weight loss is increased if the patient has a poor appetite and does not want to eat. It gives the impression that the patient is dying of malnutrition and therefore neglect. Feeding a patient is one of the few things which the carers feel competent to do, and if the patient is unable to eat, their sense of helplessness is magnified.

Causes

Cancer Related

Most cancer patients experience loss of appetite. One third will have anorexia for more than 6 months, another third for 1–6 months. Weight loss can occur with all types of cancer, but the frequency depends on the diagnosis and how long the patient has had cancer. Patients with lymphoma have the lowest incidence of weight loss (less than 50%); lung, colon and prostate cancers have an intermediate incidence (50%–60%); and gastric and pancreatic cancers produce the highest incidence (> 80%) (De Wys et al., 1980). Breast cancer patients presenting for adjuvant chemotherapy have a very low incidence (only 2%), increasing to less than half of the patients requiring treatment for first recurrence and to two-thirds of terminally ill patients.

There are many ways in which cancer patients lose weight. Head and neck cancers reduce food intake by interfering with swallowing, either by a mass effect or by neuromuscular dysfunction from damage to the cranial nerves. Oesophageal and intra-abdominal malignancies can cause bowel obstruction. Pancreatic cancer can produce malabsorption. However, direct effects do not explain weight loss in most patients. There is now considerable evidence to implicate distant paraneoplastic effects of cancer.

Despite the similar appearance of cachexia and malnutrition patients, the metabolic abnormalities are very different. Cachexia patients often have a higher metabolic rate, higher than normal in some cases, with active breakdown rather than preservation of protein stores. There are other marked differences in carbohydrate and lipid metabolism. Cytrokines have been implicated in promoting the anorexia/cachexia syndrome. Tumour necrosis factor (previously known as cachectin), and interleukins 1 (IL-1) and 6 (IL-6) are produced by cancer cells and by the body in response to the presence of cancer. They cause anorexia and weight loss in animal models (Bruera and Higginson, 1986). Recently a lipid-activating factor has also been discovered.

Treatment Related

Chemotherapy causes weight loss in several ways. Nausea and vomiting will stop patients eating. Some drugs, such as cisplatin and DTIC, are very likely to cause emesis, while drugs such as daunorubicin, doxorubicin, carmustine and procarbazine have moderate emetogenic potential. Chemotherapy-induced mouth ulceration will cause patients to avoid eating. Chemotherapy can damage the epithelial surface of the small bowel, impairing food absorption, but the clinical implications of this effect are probably minimal.

Some of the early effects of radiotherapy can cause temporary weight loss. Painful mucositis following treatment of the mouth or oesophagus can severely limit the patient's ability to eat. If the small bowel or the brainstem lie within the radiotherapy field, nausea and vomiting will have the same effect. Inflammation of the gut may produce diarrhoea and malabsorption. Long-term effects include fibrosis, stricturing, ulceration, fistula formation or perforation of the bowel. These late effects may be delayed for years when the ensuing weight loss may be mistaken for the effects of advanced cancer. The effects of radiotherapy and chemotherapy are additive.

For patients who require major gastrointestinal surgery, temporary weight loss occurs due to the removal of the tumour, fluid losses and catabolic effects. Longer lasting effects occur if swallowing is disrupted, if persistent stricture or fistulae develop, or a short-bowel syndrome is produced. Patients who have been gastrectomised become malnourished.

The effects of treatment are usually transient and the patient's weight will recover if remission is achieved. If a patient has persistent or rapidly recurrent disease, continued weight loss will occur. In the latter case, the recurrence may not be readily apparent, resulting in the patient being continually reassured that all should be well.

Prior weight loss has adverse effects on treatments. Cachectic patients do not respond as well to chemotherapy. The tolerance of cachectic patients to radio-therapy is also reduced. Patients with significant weight loss have greater mortality and morbidity from major operations.

Other Conditions

The most important non-malignant cause of weight loss is chronic bacterial infection. Abscesses can be associated with head and neck cancers, cavitating lung cancers, fungating tumours and colorectal tumours. Fevers, rigors, signs of inflammation and offensive discharge should indicate the diagnosis.

Management

Oncological Treatments

The paraneoplastic cachexia–anorexia syndrome will abate if the cancer can be treated. The specific treatment modality will depend on the type of cancer, degree of spread, and the general condition of the patient.

Other Treatments

Enteral and Parenteral Nutrition

Nutritional support has been used for cachectic patients who are receiving curative and palliative treatments. Overall, there has been no convincing evidence that this makes any difference except in patients undergoing gastro-intestinal surgery, or in patients with severe gut dysfunction who are receiving effective chemotherapy.

The use of aggressive nutritional measures is not recommended for patients with advanced cancer for whom effective anti-cancer treatment is not available. Studies have not shown any prolongation of survival. Experimental animal models have suggested that parenteral nutrition accelerates the growth of un-treated cancer. There have been anecdotal reports of similar effects in patients (Rice and Van Rij, 1987). These observations can be helpful in explaining why parenteral nutrition should not be used for patients with advanced incurable cancer. Some patients do benefit from enteral nutrition, notably patients who have some cause for malnutrition as well as cachexia. A common example is the patient with head and neck cancer who cannot swallow because of the local effects of the disease and treatment. These patients lose weight but also feel hungry, as distinct from the patients with advanced disease who are anorexic. A decision to start enteral nutrition should always be reviewed when the patient's general condition deteriorates.

Mouth Care

Aggressive mouth care and appropriate use of systemic or topical analgesics can minimise the effects of chemotherapy and radiotherapy to the mouth and oesophagus. Dose reduction of the chemotherapy agents may be necessary if stomatitis is related to neutropenia.

Antiemetics

A trial of an antiemetic drug, such as haloperidol 1.5 mg twice daily, may improve appetite in patients with cachexia, even if nausea or vomiting are not problems. The recently introduced $5HT_3$ receptor antagonists have been particularly effective in relieving the emetic effects of chemotherapy and radio-therapy.

Corticosteroids

Corticosteroids can stimulate appetite in patients with advanced cancer, pro-vided that infection and other contra-indications have been excluded. A dose of dexamethasone 4 mg daily or equivalent is usually sufficient, given in the morning. Regular injections of methylprednisolone used to be given for this indication but they are no more effective and are less convenient than the oral route. Some patients will only get partial improvement; the dose can be increased up to 16 mg per day if necessary. Once a satisfactory response has been obtained, the dose can be reduced to the lowest dose that maintains the response. Usually, patients do not survive long enough to develop the myopathic and other longer term side-effects of steroid therapy.

Progestagens

For those patients who do have a longer prognosis, the progestagens offer an alternative to steroids. High doses need to be used, such as 800 mg of medroxy-progesterone acetate daily. These doses can be given to male patients without causing nausea. Fluid retention can be a problem but usually only in patients with lymphoedema. Patients often appreciate the improvement in facial appear-ance which is normally considered a side-effect. Both steroids and progestagens have been shown to decrease levels of IL-6, one of the cytokine mediators of cachexia.

Antihistamines

Cyproheptadine is an antihistamine which has appetite-stimulating effects. It is no longer used because of the associated drowsiness.

Other Measures

While some patients appreciate the opportunity afforded by the appetite stimulants, many are satisfied with a simple explanation about the process of cachexia emphasising that the effects of cancer are not caused by malnutrition and that even parenteral nutrition would not prolong survival. Relatives are more likely to be distressed by the patient's anorexia than the patient, and they need particular reassurance. They can be advised to prepare smaller meals which are served on a small plate. This will often be more attractive to the patients thereby allaying some of the helplessness experienced by the carers.

Weakness

During the terminal phase of cancer, weakness is an almost universal symptom. A few patients die suddenly (about 2%), but the remainder experience some degree of exercise limitation. Patients use the term 'weakness' to refer to loss of muscle strength or a feeling of lassitude. Either meaning has the same end result. If weakness is severe enough, the patient will require assistance with self-care. This loss of independence can be very distressing – the ultimate loss of dignity. It can cause more suffering than physical pain.

Causes

Cancer Related

The cachexia process is associated with weakness. De Wys et al. (1980) noted that weight loss was associated with reduced performance status except in patients with pancreatic and gastric cancer. This suggests that the loss of muscle protein and other catabolic effects play an important role. Cancer-related weakness due to cachexia is a poor prognostic sign. Other causes of weakness associated with cancer include the paraneoplastic effects on muscle, such as myositis and proximal myopathy, on neuromuscular function, and on nerves producing neuropathy. Some cancers produce bone marrow failure with anaemia. A low haemoglobin will cause or exacerbate weakness. Brain tumours can produce weakness from hemipares.

Spinal cord compression is a very important cause of weakness which must be recognised early, otherwise the patient is left with permanent disability, not only paraplegia, but also double incontinence. Spinal cord compression usually results from an extradural metastatic mass which presses against the spinal cord. Reactive oedema increases the neurological deficit. Permanent neurological damage quickly follows producing the clinical signs described above. Collapse or displacement of an unstable vertebral body can suddenly transect the cord. A high index of suspicion is needed to make the diagnosis before irreversible spinal cord damage occurs.

Most patients with spinal cord compression will have had a prior history of a dull aching back pain. The pain will have been present for several days or weeks. If vertebral body collapse occurs, the pain will suddenly increase and be associated with nerve pain radiating into the dermatome. Sometimes, a sharp shooting pain will radiate into the legs. At some point, neurological symptoms and signs will occur. The patient may suddenly become paraplegic, but more usually the patient begins to experience difficulty walking, then increasing weakness and altered sensation in the legs, followed by urinary retention, loss of anal tone, and complete paraplegia. Clinical signs include upper limb and truncal weakness if the compression is high enough, lower limb spasticity and up-going plantars if the compression is above the origin of the cauda equina, and lower motor neurone leg weakness if the level is below. A sensory level, bladder distension and lax anal sphincter tone may also be present. The prognosis for recovery is determined by the disability present when treatment is commenced. Complete paraplegia with double incontinence is very unlikely to improve, hence the need to make the diagnosis before these occur.

The diagnosis of spinal cord compression is made by MRI scanning or, less commonly, CT myelography. Twenty per cent of patients will have more than one site of compression. Treatment is usually by radiotherapy. High-dose dexamethasone (at least 16 mg per day) is started when the diagnosis is suspected. Surgery may be required if there is vertebral body instability. Laminectomy alone is not sufficient because instability is often increased.

Treatment Related

Courses of radiotherapy and chemotherapy may be associated with temporary tiredness and weakness. Also, major operations often leave patients feeling weak for a time. These effects will compound any pre-existing weakness from advanced cancer. Long-term steroid use, to control raised intracranial pressure from primary and secondary brain tumours, for example, will eventually produce a disabling proximal myopathy.

Management

Oncological Treatments

As for the paraneoplastic cachexia–anorexia syndrome, weakness will improve if the cancer is treatable. However, a decision to start treatment must be balanced against the poor prognosis and the difficulties patients will have tolerating the treatment.

Other Treatments

Blood Transfusion
Weak patients may improve with a blood transfusion if the haemoglobin level is less than 9 g/l. If the patient appears to have advanced disease, the choice of trying a transfusion should be made in discussion with the patient. In this situation, a transfusion of no more than two units should be given very slowly to prevent fluid overload. Often the patient will decline the option.

Corticosteroids
A trial of steroids may be warranted if a patient is anguished by weakness. Dexamethasone 4–16 mg in the morning may produce an improvement in energy levels as well as appetite. Steroids may occasionally help the paraneoplastic effects of cancer on nerves and muscles.

Physiotherapy

Physiotherapists can help patients to adapt to progressive weakness. A modified exercise routine can provide psychological as well as physical improvement. Patients can also be advised how to pace activities within their current energy reserves.

Psychological Support

In practice, even if the above measures work, they only delay the inevitable decline. Patients who cannot accept the progressive weakness will need a lot of psychological support, as will their families. The approach to managing anguish is outlined in the chapter on spiritual pain.

Delirium

Delirium is a relatively common event in people who are terminally ill. It is characterised by reduced awareness of the environment and disordered cognition. The latter manifests itself as disorientation in person, time and place. The patient often appears bewildered, has disordered thoughts and performs inappropriate actions. Occasionally, patients will be aware of their confusion and become more distressed. Other patients become agitated as part of the delirium, experiencing hallucinations and delusions. They may develop insomnia, day-night reversal, increased motor activity, such as picking at bed clothes, and begin shouting or crying out.

Confusion and delirium can be very upsetting for families. They often describe 'losing' the patient, as if he or she is already dead. The sense of impending loss is heightened by the sense of helplessness.

The sudden onset of confusion suggests delirium, also known as acute brain syndrome. A treatable cause should be sought because the confusion may be reversible. A chronic confusional state suggests dementia. These patients have a history of progressive memory loss, which may be associated with personality change and nocturnal restlessness. Cancer is more common in the age group in which dementia is likely. Patients with early dementia will tip more easily into a severe confusional state when exposed to the factors which cause delirium.

Assessment of Delirium

Delirium is multifactorial encompassing physical, emotional and spiritual factors. A thorough assessment is needed. If a patient presents as confused, the carers should be asked when the confusion started. This should establish if the problem is acute or chronic. It is important to know about any new changes in medication, clinical condition or mental state which might have precipitated the confusional state or made a pre-existing problem worse. Careful clinical examination may reveal an underlying infection, signs of hepatic or renal failure, cyanosis or evidence of cerebral metastases. Routine biochemical tests may further define the cause. Other tests, such as chest x-ray, may be appropriate, depending on the clinical findings. Restless patients who are dying should not be subjected to investigations. A clinical assessment will often be all that is necessary to exclude the important treatable causes.

Causes

Cancer Related

Confusion is often attributed to cerebral metastases. In practice, this is rarely the case. Other causes of confusion should be excluded before this diagnosis is made. Some deep-seated or frontal lobe cerebral tumours may cause a confusional state but other neurological features will usually be present. Occasionally, a tumour will cause a nominal aphasia where the patient cannot name objects. This can be interpreted as confusion until the content of the conversation is recognised as normal.

There are two important metabolic syndromes associated with cancer which can produce delirium: hypercalcaemia and hyponatraemia. Hypercalcaemia is relatively common. It is found with breast and lung cancer, multiple myeloma, lymphoma, melanoma, squamous cell carcinomas of the head and neck, and prostate cancer. Confusion usually occurs when the patient becomes dehydrated from the salt and fluid losses through the kidneys. This also results in the symptoms of thirst and polyuria. The other symptoms include drowsiness, nausea and constipation. A dehydrated patient with hypercalcaemia may look as if he or she is dying. The gaunt appearance and drowsiness are very similar. Hypercalcaemia is suggested when the deterioration is sudden, the patient is thirsty and continues to be incontinent of urine when no longer able to drink. Dying patients usually stop being thirsty and stop passing urine.

Hyponatraemia is associated with small cell lung cancer. Inappropriate levels of antidiuretic hormone are produced which cause water retention. Salt excretion by the kidneys is normal so that peripheral oedema is not a feature. The patient develops signs of water 'intoxication' with confusion resulting from neuronal dysfunction. As with hypercalcaemia, the deterioration is relatively sudden. The physical appearance of the patient is unchanged.

Cancer patients are more susceptible to infections, especially when the disease is advanced. Chest and urinary-tract infections are common, but pressure sores may become a site of infection if pressure-area care is not maintained.

Hepatic failure from liver metastases or primary hepatocellular carcinoma will produce confusion. This is a very late manifestation and usually a sign that the patient is dying. The patient will often be jaundiced and will have a flapping tremor. The ammonia-like smell on the patient's breath is another characteristic sign.

Severe hypoxia, usually associated with lung cancer and chest infection, will induce confusion. The patient may appear cyanosed and tachypnoeic. Arterial blood gas analysis will establish the diagnosis. A pulse oximeter is less traumatic and can be used in a hospice.

Severe psychological distress, for example, fear of impending death or the prospect of uncontrolled pain, or the prior use of denial to cope with the diagnosis, will exacerbate delirium and make the patient very agitated.

Treatment Related

Cranial irradiation can produce a delayed reaction which may be associated with confusion some weeks after treatment. The reaction is transient and settles without treatment. However, the delayed onset may precipitate a mistaken diagnosis of deterioration due to disease progression.

Patients receiving chemotherapy can develop severe infection, particularly if they are neutropenic. The first sign of sepsis may be delirium, caused by the infection itself and hypotension. Some of these patients may be under the care of a hospice home-care service. It is important that the possibility of infection is considered and acted upon if the hospice service is first contacted by the patient or family. Failure to recognise this complication can result in the rapid deterioration and death of the patient.

Several drugs used in palliative care will cause delirium. The elderly are more prone, as are patients with liver and renal dysfunction, depending on how the drug is metabolised and cleared. Morphine can cause a toxic confusional state, often associated with myoclonic jerking. NSAIDs are commonly used as analgesics, but are only rarely implicated as a cause of confusion, as are the H_2 blockers such as cimetidine. Corticosteroids can precipitate a paranoid psychosis which is idiosyncratic. This side-effect does not only occur at higher doses. Hyoscine is widely used to dry secretions, treat colic and control nausea. Elderly patients can experience confusion and psychosis with the hydrobromide salt, which is why hyoscine butylbromide or glycopyrronium are preferred.

Other Conditions

Atherosclerotic cerebrovascular disease can cause stroke which is sometimes associated with confusion. The confusion will happen suddenly and there should be other signs of neurological deficit. Alcohol, benzodiazepine and barbiturate withdrawal are all potential problems, especially when patients become too ill to swallow. Many hospice in-patient units routinely offer patients alcohol, partly to avoid withdrawal symptoms in those who are alcohol dependent.

Drugs used to treat other illnesses may cause delirium when the patient deteriorates. There are many examples, but one common problem relates to hypoglycaemic agents. The insulin requirements of diabetic patients often fall as the illness progresses, unless steroid therapy is needed. If long-acting oral agents or insulins are continued, the risk of significant hypoglycaemia increases. Tight control of blood glucose levels are not appropriate. Most patients should be converted to shorter-acting preparations or have current doses reduced as anorexia increases.

Management

General Measures

There are several general steps which should be considered before medications are started. The distress associated with delirium may be minimised if the patient is cared for in quiet bright surroundings. The home will be the most familiar environment for the patient, but the most difficult for the family. If the patient needs admission, the family should be encouraged to stay with the patient. However, they may be exhausted and need a rest.

Every opportunity should be taken to orientate the patient gently, with reminders about where the patient is, and what day and what time it is. This information should be communicated in a matter-of-fact, not a demeaning, manner. Familiar objects, photographs and pets may help. Spectacles and hearing aids should be worn if the patient normally uses them.

Corticosteroids

A trial of high-dose steroids may be warranted if cerebral metastases are suspected, bearing in mind that steroids may increase agitation from other causes. Steroids may also be tried if confusion occurs after intracranial radiotherapy.

Correcting Metabolic Disturbances

Intravenous rehydration and bisphosphonates will improve confusion due to hypercalcaemia. Some patients will maintain lower levels of serum calcium for several weeks after a single does. The effect usually takes two or three days. More rapid reduction of calcium is possible with calcitonin. Mithramycin is no longer used. If high levels of parathormone-like activity are present, the calcium level will rise after two or three weeks and repeat doses of bisphosphanate will be needed. Regular doses of an orally active bisphosphanate can be given. Oral phosphate can also be effective, but the dose has to titrated carefully to prevent diarrhoea.

Hyponatraemia will respond to severe water restriction (no more than 500 ml per day) and oral demeclocycline.

Antibiotics

The use of antibiotics to treat infection will depend on the general condition of the patient. Severe infection in an otherwise well patient will require intravenous treatment. The decision to start treatment in a terminally ill patient must be taken very carefully. If the patient is well enough to take oral medications and the confusion is likely to recover or the patient still has unfinished business to complete, a trial may be worthwhile. If treatment is successful, the delirium may be slow to lift. Generally, however, infection marks the final event in the illness and antibiotics only prove troublesome to administer.

Oxygen

Hypoxia associated with confusion is an indication for oxygen therapy. Administration via nasal prongs is often sufficient. Care must be taken if hypercapnia is likely.

Drug-Induced Confusion

Any drugs suspected of creating problems should be stopped if possible. If the drug is still necessary, for example, a strong opioid for pain, then the dose should be lowered or a change made to an alternative analgesic. Where a choice of drugs is available, for example, the anticholinergic drugs, the preparation least likely to penetrate the blood–brain barrier should be used.

Major Tranquillisers and Sedatives

The use of major tranquillisers and sedatives should be integrated into a broader plan of action. Too often the temptation is to start sedatives without checking for reversible causes and without assessing the psychological state. If these factors are not considered, sedatives may worsen the problem by increasing the patient's distress at being out of control. Some patients do not even require sedatives. They will remain pleasantly muddled and the response to the treatment of reversible causes can be awaited.

If treatment is needed for mild confusion and distress, a low dose of a major tranquilliser is preferable to a benzodiazepine. Haloperidol 2.5–5 mg twice daily or thioridazine 12.5–25 mg two or three times daily may ease the situation without producing drowsiness. The dose can be gradually increased if necessary. Supplementary doses of diazepam (2 mg every 6–8 mg) may help if anxiety is a feature. Chlorpromazine is more likely to precipitate symptomatic hypotension and drowsiness.

Confused patients who are very agitated need to be settled quickly. Medications are almost always needed. Attempts to calm the patient with rational discussion usually make the agitation worse. Parenteral drugs should be given. Midazolam 10 mg can be injected subcutaneously and will cause sedation within minutes. This can be followed up with a major tranquilliser such as haloperidol 10–20 mg or methotrimeprazine 25–50 mg. Sometimes the patient will be more settled on awakening, allowing maintenance treatment to be given orally. Otherwise, repeated injections will be needed and the patient will have to be kept sedated. This is always a difficult outcome. The family will need to be kept informed but the decision should not be devolved to them lest they be left with an unacceptable burden of guilt.

The use of sedation raises several important ethical issues. The patient may be too confused to consent to treatment. Worse still, the extremely agitated patient may resist treatment which can then only be given forcibly. If the agitation does not settle with the initial treatment or with treatment of reversible causes, sedation may have to be continued, putting the patient at risk of developing pneumonia. These issues are considered in more detail in the chapter on ethics.

Terminal Restlessness

Terminal restlessness is a state of physical restlessness which occurs when some patients are dying. Whereas most patients lie quietly, exhausted by the physical effects of the cancer, restlessness is characterised by semi-purposeful movements such as attempts to sit or get out of bed, plucking at the air or bed clothes, and constant efforts to change position in the bed. Some restlessness patients are confused, many are too weak to answer questions.

Causes

Many of the causes of delirium will also produce restlessness when a patient is dying. However, it will not be appropriate to investigate or specifically treat these causes. Dying patients who become restless may be experiencing discomfort. Pain may only be obvious from non-verbal signs such as grimacing and vocalising. Urinary retention and faecal impaction should also be considered as correctable causes of restlessness.

Continued steroid therapy will produce restlessness when the body is no longer able to respond to the therapeutic effects. Once the patient has lost the improvement in appetite or energy provided by a palliative course of steroids, the dose should be decreased.

Occasionally, patients who have denied their terminal illness become very agitated and restless when they lose the strength to maintain the denial. This will also happen if a patient becomes very fearful in the final stages, for example, at the prospect of impending death.

Management

General Measures

Every effort should be made to rule out the easily treated causes of terminal restlessness. Sometimes, the tendency is just to increase the dose of morphine, but a urinary catheter will be much more effective in treating urinary retention, for example. A dying patient who becomes frightened will usually need medication to relax, but a staff member sitting with the patient will bring reassurance and extra comfort. The importance of reducing or stopping steroids has already been highlighted.

NSAIDs

Dying patients can become very sensitive to skin pressure and touch. They will be uncomfortable if turned. If an NSAID is not already being used, regular suppositories (for example, diclofenac 100 mg twice daily) or injections (for example, diclofenac 75 mg twice daily or ketorolac 15 mg six hourly) should be tried. Topical application of an NSAID can be effective for painful pressure sores, though prevention is best.

Opioids

Additional doses of morphine may be needed for pain or breathlessness. Morphine should not be used as a sedative. It is not as effective as drugs designed for this purpose and may cause excitatory effects such as jerking and twitching if given in higher doses than are needed for pain.

Benzodiazepines

Midazolam and flunitrazepam are very useful for relieving terminal restlessness. Small doses can be given subcutaneously (for example, midazolam 2.5–5 mg) at 15 minute intervals until the patient is settled. Respiratory depression is not a problem. Regular doses can be continued, usually as a continuous infusion via a syringe driver.

Major Tranquillisers

Methotrimeprazine is often used for terminal restlessness, either singly or in combination with midazolam. It can be given subcutaneously at a dose of 25–50 mg every 6–8 hours or via a syringe driver.

Dry Mouth

Dry mouth is a symptom that is often missed. It makes swallowing difficult and induces a constant need to drink.

Causes

Cancer Related

Dying patients often give up drinking. This leads to concerns about dehydration, but surprisingly, dry mouth is not a common complaint from these patients.

Ellershaw et al. (1995) showed that dry mouth and thirst were not associated with biochemical signs of dehydration.

Treatment Related

Radiotherapy to the head and neck will cause mouth dryness if the salivary glands are treated. This can be very disabling to patients who already have difficulty swallowing after surgery. The lack of saliva has other important consequences for dental hygiene. Gum disease and dental caries are more likely. These patients should have regular dental follow-up from someone who is experienced in managing these complications following radiotherapy

Medications are the commonest cause of dry mouth in the terminally ill. Elderly patients are especially prone. It is a well recognised side-effect of the anticholinergic drugs which are frequently used in palliative care, such as amitriptyline for pain, and hyoscine for colic, nausea and secretions. Morphine can also cause mouth dryness.

Other Conditions

Occasionally, oral thrush will be associated with mouth dryness. The mouth will appear red and inflamed; plaque will not necessarily be evident. The mouth dryness may not be caused by the thrush, but it will increase any other symptoms, such as mouth soreness.

Management

Symptomatic Treatments

General Measures
Patients who have mouth dryness post-radiotherapy should have a programme of oral mouth cares. Drugs which cause or exacerbate mouth dryness should be stopped or substituted. Dying patients can be managed by being given small sips of fluid or chips of ice to suck. Offering drinks of fluid is usually not helpful. The patient may feel compelled to take a drink, only to aspirate because of the lack of strength and co-ordination. Family members can be taught how to wet a mouth swab and place it carefully to the patient's lips. This gives them something positive to do during this difficult time.

Artificial Saliva
There are several artificial saliva preparations commercially available in liquid or spray from. Mixtures can also be made up by pharmacists. Glycerine-based products should be avoided. Some patients find the products based on methyl-cellulose to be extremely helpful but others have no benefit.

Antifungal Agents

A trial of nystatin or miconazole is warranted if thrush is suspected.

Pilocarpine

Recent reports have highlighted the benefit of the muscarinic cholinergic agonist pilocarpine, particularly for patients with radiotherapy-induced dry mouth. If the dose is carefully titrated, side-effects are minimal.

Tumour Fungation

Malignant tumours which penetrate the skin or mucous membranes often necrose and ulcerate. The cosmetic distress of rapidly growing unsightly lesions is made worse if infection occurs. Anaerobic bacteria will produce an unpleasant odour, discharge and bleeding. Haemorrhage can also occur from tumour-related vessels within the lesion or from erosion of adjacent arteries. Bleeding from the latter can cause exsanguination.

Causes

Cancer Related

Fungation occurs with breast cancer, head and neck tumours, and skin and lymph node metastases from melanoma and squamous cell skin tumours. Colon cancers can invade through the abdominal wall. Vulval and anal cancers are uncommon, but local spread and lymph node fungation is the more distressing because of the location.

Treatment Related

Skin ulceration can occur as a late effect of radiotherapy. The ulcer lacks the rolled edge of a malignant ulcer. Fortunately, this side-effect is very rare but may still be found in some patients who had radical treatment for breast carcinoma several years ago. If radiotherapy is used to treat a skin lesion, fungation may occur as tumour necrosis takes place. The skin will heal over if the cancer is destroyed.

Management

Oncological Treatments

All of the anti-cancer treatment modalities may have a role in controlling fungating wounds, depending on the primary diagnosis and previous treatment.

Unfortunately, active treatments may only have a temporary effect. The side-effects of radiation may exacerbate skin problems in the treatment phase.

Other Treatments

Dressings
Dressings are the mainstay of treatment for lesions which cannot be removed or cured. They serve a cosmetic function and soak up any discharge. A wide range of absorbent dressings is now available. Non-stick dressings are best for open wounds. Some dressings contain charcoal which will absorb odour. Large fungating wounds may need several dressings joined together for coverage.

Antibiotics
Antibiotics with anaerobic cover will control smell and discharge. They may also be useful in reducing bleeding from infected lesions. Some patients need antibiotics to control systemic symptoms of infection from fungating wounds.

Haemostatic Measures
If bleeding is a recurrent or severe problem, swabs soaked in adrenaline solution can be applied. A more expensive option is topical thrombin. When major arteries are threatened, ligation or embolisation may be possible if other organs will not be compromised.

Somatostatin Analogues
Fungating colorectal tumours can produce a profuse watery or mucous discharge. This can be reduced with octreotide. It must be given by subcutaneous infusion, starting at 100 mcg daily, increasing to 600 mcg daily.

Fistulae

Cancers have the potential to erode through normal body tissues creating fistulae. These allow bodily fluids and malignant discharges to issue from abnormal connections. This can be extremely distressing, as with the constant leakage of faeces from a recto-vaginal fistula or from a fistulous connection between the colon and skin. Bladder fistulae produce the indignity of urinary incontinence and the discomfort of skin excoriation.

Causes

Cancer Related

Pelvic and intra-abdominal tumours, such as colorectal and cervical cancer, produce vesicorectal, vesicovaginal, rectovaginal, enterocolic and enterocutaneous fistulae. The other common potential site for fistula formation is the head and neck. A fistula between the mouth and skin, for example, will add a discharge of saliva to the disfigurement of the tumour and previous treatment. Oesophageal and lung cancers may produce tracheo-oesophageal fistulae.

Treatment Related

Fistula formation is a recognised complication of bowel and other surgical operations

Successful treatment of locally advanced pelvic or head and neck tumours with radiotherapy and chemotherapy may cause a fistula as the cancer is destroyed. If previous surgery has been used, it can be difficult to decide whether the fistula is related to tumour recurrence or tumour destruction. Scarring around the fistula may mask histological recurrence.

Rarely, fistulae may form as a late effect of radiotherapy. A patient treated with external beam and intracavitatory radiotherapy for carcinoma of the cervix might develop a vesico-vaginal fistula many years later. Extensive fibrosis will again make it difficult to exclude recurrence.

Management

Surgical Repair/Bypass

If a benign cause for a fistula is confirmed, surgical repair or bypass is the best solution. Intricate operations have been devised using omentum to repair post-radiotherapy vesicovaginal fistulae, for example.

Malignant fistulae involving bowel should also be treated with bypass procedures. This usually requires colostomy formation but occasionally an entero-enterostomy will obviate the need for a stoma. Urinary diversion procedures can help patients with bladder fistulae if the prognosis is more than a few months. Surgical attempts at local treatment of large active malignant fistulae are fraught with problems. Temporary relief may be obtained, but the symptoms are often made worse.

Stomatherapist

A good stomatherapist is invaluable in providing advice about appliances and other measures to help minimise the impact on patients' quality of life. Their expertise should be involved as soon as possible in the management process. Stoma appliances can be adapted to fit over discharging fistulae in many unusual and awkward sites.

Somatostatin Analogues

Patients with faecal fistulae who refuse surgery or who have multiple inoperable lesions can have good symptomatic improvement with continuous infusions of octreotide (100–600 mcg daily). This will reduce the volume and consistency of the discharge to levels that are manageable with stoma appliances. This is especially helpful with high-volume small-bowel fistulae that would otherwise require parenteral nutrition for control.

Urinary Catheter

The urinary incontinence of small but troublesome bladder fistulae may be effectively controlled by an indwelling catheter. This may have to be introduced by the suprapubic route if there is extensive tumour involving the urethra and introitus.

Vasopressin

Synthetic antidiuretic hormone analogues can be used to reduce urinary output and therefore incontinence if a catheter or other means of urinary diversion is not possible. Vasopressin nasal spray offers a convenient method of administration. This is best used for nocturnal incontinence which is the most distressing. Otherwise the patient may develop water intoxication.

Anticholinergic Drugs

Mucocutaneous fistulae involving the mouth will lose large quantities of saliva. Patients have to wear absorbent towels and bibs which need frequent changing. Clothes become soaked with the discharge. A regular dose of an anticholinergic drug may make a big difference. The transdermal hyoscine patches are convenient and give a constant blood level. They need only be changed every three days. Sometimes, two patches are needed at the same time.

Itch

Itch is uncommon but potentially very troublesome. If it is severe enough, sleep will be disrupted and the patient may develop bleeding from the scratch marks. Although the sensation of itch is probably transmitted in pain fibres, routine analgesics are not effective.

Causes

Cancer Related

Obstructive jaundice is a potent cause of itch. The itch may occur as the earliest symptom, possibly as a result of bile salt deposition in the skin. Carcinoma of the pancreas, ampulla of water or cholangiocarcinomas, will all obstruct the biliary tree. Widespread intrahepatic disease may produce the same effect. Patients with advanced lymphomas, particularly Hodgkin's, can develop pruritis in association with other systemic symptoms such as fevers and sweats. Other haematological malignancies which cause itch include leukaemia and polycythaemia rubra vera. Pruritis is a feature of renal failure, which can be caused by pelvic cancers in particular.

Treatment Related

Drug allergy should always be considered if a rash is also present. Some drugs such as chlorpromazine may precipitate cholestatic jaundice. Itch is sometimes associated with morphine therapy. It is more common when morphine is given by the epidural route.

Other Causes

Inflammatory pancreatic disease can mimic carcinoma of the pancreas. This possibility must always be borne in mind, even though a histological diagnosis of pancreatic carcinoma may have been made. Patients with pre-existing skin disease will present with itch.

Management

General Measures

Patients who are troubled by itch should wear cool light garments. Heat should be avoided, for example, hot showers will make itch worse. Physical means, such as cotton gloves, should be used to help the patient stop scratching. Moisturisers and soap substitutes which do not contain lanolin can be soothing.

Oncological Treatments

Most causes of malignant obstructive jaundice cannot be treated actively. Bypass surgery was often used before the introduction of biliary stents. The operation had the advantage that a gastro-jejunostomy could be performed at the same time. However, the mortality and morbidity from these procedures is high.

Chemotherapy options are often considered for lymphoma patients even after first and second relapse. Symptomatic control may be best achieved with palliative chemotherapy.

Other Treatments

Biliary Stenting
The use of biliary stents has dramatically decreased the problem of itch from obstructive jaundice. They are easily placed into the common bile duct via an endoscope. Sometimes, a cannula has to be inserted percutaneously. Stents last several months and may need to be replaced. Ascending cholangitis can occur but is rarely life threatening. It can make the patient appear to be deteriorating from the cancer, except that the change is more sudden and there will be fevers and rigors. Broad-spectrum oral antibiotics are often satisfactory to control this if the stent cannot be changed.

Antihistamines
Antihistamines have long been recommended for pruritis. Topical applications should be avoided as they may produce further skin sensitisation. Oral antihistamines frequently have a sedative effect which may, in part, explain their usefulness. While this effect may be helpful at night, few patients appreciate the 'hung-over' feeling during the day. Consequently, a non-sedating antihistamine such as terfenadine would be the drug of choice for daytime use. An H_2 receptor blocker such as cimetidine can be used in combination.

Sedatives
Other sedative drugs are sometimes used to reduce itch and scratching at night. Phenothiazines have been recommended, but a trial of a benzodiazepine may be worthwhile.

Cholestyramine
Cholestyramine is an ion-exchange resin which binds bile salts in the gut. The starting dose is 4 g daily, increasing up to 24 g daily. However, it is very unpalatable and few terminally ill patients can tolerate the taste even if it is disguised. It also causes constipation and bowel softeners are essential.

5-HT₃ Receptor Antagonists
Ondansetron has been used successfully to treat the itch of obstructive jaundice. It is an expensive medication that should not be considered 'first line'.

Androgenic Steroids
The use of androgenic steroids such as methyltestosterone has been recommended if the above measures fail.

Rifampicin
The antituberculous drug rifampicin can relieve itch in patients with primary biliary cirrhosis. The authors have no experience of this drug in patients with malignant biliary obstruction.

Bile Acid Solvents
There is a group of drugs which are used to dissolve gallstones. Ursodeoxycholic acid is one example which can be given orally and has been effective for some patients with cholestatis from malignant obstruction. These drugs are expensive and can cause gastrointestinal upset.

Convulsions

Generalised convulsions may cause few symptoms for patients. They may be aware of a prodrome but more often they find themselves recovering from a fit with no recollection of what happened. However, any family who witnesses a generalised seizure will be very distressed and may refuse to care for the patient at home. Patients are more likely to experience the effects of partial seizures when loss of consciousness does not occur. The uncontrollable shaking of a limb involved in a Jacksonian fit or the unpleasant emotions aroused by a temporal lobe fit can be distressing to the patient.

If convulsions are suspected, a careful history should be taken from any observers. The nature and circumstances of the event should be noted in detail. Fainting episodes can be misinterpreted as fits, for example, resulting in patients having to take long-term medications unnecessarily. Occasionally, the expertise of a neurologist may be required to establish the diagnosis. A CT head scan or MRI scan should be considered in those patients who do not have known intracerebral disease.

Causes

Cancer Related

Primary and secondary brain tumours are both associated with fits. A convulsion may be the first manifestation of intracerebral disease. Some histological types have a higher propensity, for example, oligodendrogliomas.

Treatment Related

Surgery and radiotherapy do not reduce the risk of further fits in patients with brain tumours. If the treatment is successful, structural brain damage will still remain as a possible trigger point. Surgery to the brain may increase the possibility of fits. Several drugs used in palliative care can lower seizure threshold. They should be avoided or only used with caution in patients with epilepsy. Examples include tricyclic antidepressants, phenothiazines, antihistamines, and anticholinergic drugs such as hyoscine. Very high doses of morphine can have a neuroexcitatory effect.

Other Conditions

A variety of other diseases will precipitate seizures. Severe hypoxia, infection and renal failure can all occur in terminally ill patients. Postural hypotension can simulate a seizure if a patient loses consciousness and is not laid down.

Management

Anticonvulsants

First seizures often occur outside hospitals or hospices. By the time the patient is admitted, the fit has usually stopped. A prolonged seizure lasting more than 5–10 minutes should be stopped with medication, either diazepam 10 mg rectally or midazolam 5–10 mg by subcutaneous injections. Family members can often be taught how to administer rectal diazepam at home in the event of further fits. Their confidence will also be increased if they are taught how to position the patient and if they are given a contact telephone number. Otherwise, carers will be left frightened that the patient might die during an event which looks so terrifying.

If the fit was not associated with some acute toxic event, and a structural cause such as a brain tumour is present, prophylactic anticonvulsant therapy should be started. Phenytoin can be given as loading dose followed by a regular maintenance dose for motor seizures. Other frequently used options, especially for complex seizures, include carbamazepine and sodium valproate. The aim of treatment is to stop all seizure activity if possible. In practice, this may prove very difficult. If one drug seems to be inadequate, the dose should be increased to the maximum recommended dose, using blood levels as a guide for checking to see whether new symptoms are caused by possible toxicity. Multi-drug treatment may be necessary but should be embarked on after consultation with a specialist.

When patients who have been taking anticonvulsants begin to die, they are often unable to continue oral medications. Phenytoin and carbamazepine can be made up in suppository form and continued by the rectal route. Alternatively, diazepam can be kept handy for emergency use. A continuous infusion of midazolam or clonazepam can be considered.

Patients who develop seizures when they are dying present special problems. Subcutaneous midazolam may be sufficient but the anticonvulsant effects tend to wear off in the same way that diazepam does. Longer-acting parenteral anticonvulsants such as clonazepam (2–10 mg per day) or phenobarbitone (200–2000 mg per day) can be given by subcutaneous infusion.

Corticosteroids

Steroid therapy is often used to manage raised intracranial pressure. Anecdotally, this can help to reduce the frequency of fits. Steroids are not normally thought of as anticonvulsants and the effect may be an indirect one. However, there is some evidence that steroids do have membrane-stabilising properties.

Summary

A range of other symptoms have been considered in this chapter. Any new symptom must be taken seriously and should be carefully assessed to determine the cause. Appropriate treatments can then be started. Patients' and family members' fears and needs for information about any symptoms should always be addressed. If a symptom occurs which is not covered in this book or the recommended treatments are not effective, advice should be sought from a specialist cancer or palliative-care service.

6 – Psycho-Social Care

Introduction

In palliative medicine, psycho-social needs are considered just as important as physical symptoms. The patient and the family constitute the 'unit' of care. Each person in the family will have needs which must be recognised and met. The psychological and social issues which confront cancer patients and their families can be more significant than the physical symptoms.

The variety of psychological responses observed in palliative care were outlined in Chapter 1. Many of these responses, such as anxiety, depression and anger, will be evident from the time of diagnosis onwards. The previous chapters on symptom control in this book have highlighted some of the psychological problems that are directly related to physical symptoms. This chapter will focus on two further areas that are particularly relevant to palliative care: multicultural issues and bereavement care. The specific problems of spiritual care and suffering are covered in Chapter 7.

Multicultural Issues and Palliative Care

Hospices have existed in many countries for several decades. Before the emergence of the modern hospice movement in the 1960s, hospices were strongly associated with Christian religious orders. Although modern hospices are rarely founded and administered in this way, the association of hospices with white, middle-class Christian values has persisted, if not in reality, then certainly in the minds of health-care professionals and the public. The majority of professionals and volunteers who work in hospices are white and middle class. The common practice of naming hospices after saints reinforces the religious associations. For some patients and families, these perceived links are very important. They find that admission to a hospice is made easier by associations that are familiar and comforting. Many other patients find these same links to be unfamiliar, worrying, and even threatening.

There is good cause for hospices to be concerned about cultural issues. A recently published survey by the National Council for Hospice and Specialist Palliative Care Services (1995) highlighted how few patients from minority ethnic groups use specialist hospice services. The problem was most noticeable in hospices serving areas with a high proportion of people from minority ethnic groups. While the under-representation seems most pronounced for in-patient units, it also applies to home-care and hospital-based teams as well. Some factors for this low uptake were identified. There are fewer people from ethnic minorities in the age ranges that are associated with the highest prevalence of cancer. Some older first-generation immigrants return to their country of birth when they are terminally ill. For some minority ethnic groups, the pattern of illness is different, with a higher proportion of deaths from non-malignant conditions. Many patients and families are not aware of the existence of specialist palliative-care services. Those people who do hear about hospices are often concerned about the explicit association with death and dying. The general practitioners often come from the same ethnic group as the patients. They are also concerned about the negative connotations of hospices and are less likely to refer patients.

If palliative care is to be relevant to minority ethnic groups, a greater understanding of cultural issues is needed. Patients and families exist as part of a wider cultural set and the cultural perspective must be borne in mind when interpreting and responding to their needs. Health-care professionals are also influenced by their own cultural backgrounds. If these influences are not acknowledged, conflicts will arise and care will be jeopardised. An understanding of culture is required to appreciate these influences.

What is Culture?

Culture refers to the norms, values, beliefs and ways of behaving which characterise groups of people. The effects of culture are most visible on travelling to another country. The language, clothing, architecture and art will express the distinctive nature of the majority population. These outward signs will be accompanied by a variety of customs, rituals and implicit rules for living and relating. The purpose of culture is to provide a cohesive force enabling communities to function.

Culture also provides explanations for the various stages of human experience. Birth, rites of passage, marriage and death are given special meaning. Cultural practices help people come to terms with the impact of death and tragedy. The perceptions, explanations and rituals associated with death help to minimise anxiety, facilitate the expression of grief in an accepted way and strengthen the sense of group identity at a time when it is most threatened. Because culture is vital to the identity of any group, the transmission of cultural values is very important. Explicit teachings will be passed on by parents, grandparents, religious advisors and others. However, many cultural norms are acquired implicitly. People may only become aware of these norms when someone in the group exhibits alternative or deviant behaviour.

Cultural-norm structures exercise a powerful effect on relationships, ensuring the integrity of the group. These norms are also important for the self-esteem of each individual in the group. Self-esteem derives from a knowledge of cultural values and the ability to live according to those values. Cultural values are powerfully enforced by the reactions to deviation. If an individual breaks the norms, attempts will be made to help the person conform again. Failing this, the person will be rejected, even to the extent of being cast out. In some circumstances, the person may be ritually punished in a public demonstration.

Given that culture is important for group cohesion and personal self-esteem, a variety of strategies will be evoked when a cultural group is threatened by a different group (Solomon et al., 1995). Genocide is the worst example. Fortunately, the usual reaction is much less dramatic. Commonly, groups cope by perceiving 'outsiders' as weak, inferior and therefore less threatening. The dominant culture may attempt to reinforce these perceptions by introducing discriminatory practices, making it difficult to get jobs, housing, and education. Discrimination may be explicit but often it is covert. With time, attempts will be made to assimilate the alternative culture. Sometimes, aspects of the other culture will be accommodated into the mainstream, for example, the adoption of 'western' style clothing and music into many countries.

Culture and the Health-Care Professional

Professional care-givers need to be aware of their own cultural perspectives when working with patients and families. These perspectives will influence the behaviours of care-givers at the personal, as well as at the professional, level. Frequently, the two levels will overlap. For example, assumptions about 'right' and 'wrong' attitudes or behaviours will often be implicit, unrecognised consciously. These assumptions will have been inculcated at a personal level over many years, well before professional training. Patients or families who manifest 'wrong' behaviours may trigger anger or rejection which then clouds clinical judgement. It is unusual for such strong negative emotions to be expressed openly. Rather, health-care professionals distance themselves, for example, spending less time with the patient in clinic or visiting less often at home. It is possible this is why black and other minority ethnic groups were less likely to have adequate analgesia in the study reported by Cleeland et al. (1994).

Any tendency for health-care professionals to distance themselves from people from other cultures will be exacerbated by working with the terminally ill. One of the functions of culture is to protect people from the impact of death and dying. If individuals are made more aware of death, they become more vigorous in rejecting deviation from their cultural norms. Solomon et al. (1995) showed that experimental subjects who are exposed to videos containing material about death and dying react more aggressively towards situations and people from other cultures. The subjects' reactions occurred at a subconscious level. This work has very important implications for health-care professionals who practice in the fields of oncology and palliative medicine. The care of patients and families from minority ethnic groups must be addressed explicitly, identifying and dealing with stereotypes and prejudices that interfere with care.

In their experiments, Solomon et al. (1995) found that the effects of death awareness could be countered by providing high levels of support and praise. Enhancing self-esteem improves carers' abilities to tolerate threatening situations. Effective teamwork in palliative care has to be based on mutual support. Professionals have to overcome the usual tendency to criticise and never to give praise. Whereas many carers expect to perform their jobs without reward, palliative-care practitioners must constantly seek ways of encouraging each other.

Attitudes of Other Cultures Towards Death and Dying

There are so many different attitudes towards death and dying, even within the same culture, that it is not possible to list them all. The palliative-care literature contains several papers summarising the perspectives of specific cultural and religious groups. Some specific examples will highlight why health-care professionals need to be aware of these differences.

For many cultures, the whole concept of illness is different from the scientific medical approach that is taken for granted by lay people in Western cultures. Traditionally, there is often no concept of cancer as a specific entity; many languages do not have a word for cancer. The symptoms of cancer may not be seen as an integrated whole but may represent different illnesses. For example, a Polynesian patient with bladder cancer causing nausea, bone pain and associated nerve pain was thought by his family to have three distinct problems that were unrelated. Some people view cancer as contagious or as a sign of punishment. Many people fail to associate the systemic effects of cancer, such as weight loss and drowsiness, with the disease. This causes distress as the patient eats less and less, culminating in profound anguish when the patient stops eating and drinking.

The traditional palliative-care concept of acceptance of dying often does not hold with other cultures. Death may be seen as appropriate for some individuals, particularly the elderly. However, there may be a fear that even contemplating the death of the person will actually bring it to pass. Many cultures emphasise the need to be positive, to fight the illness, never to 'accept' what is happening, right up to the very last moment of life. This approach can cause serious conflict with palliative-care practitioners who wish to enforce a philosophy of resignation. For the families, the advice of the health-care professional will seem like complicity to murder. The distress caused to the family may be so great that they prefer to have the dying patient suffer unrelieved pain rather than have contact with the palliative-care team.

The fear of accepting death may be coupled with a fear of expressing, or even acknowledging, any powerful negative emotion such as anticipatory grief. This fear is not just based on the need to protect the patient but can be a cultural norm in other highly emotive situations. 'Bad' news, such as the diagnosis of cancer, will be withheld or modified to prevent the recipient from becoming too distressed and to prevent the family from having to deal with the distressed patient. Even if the patient is not told, the family may express their grief as anger, usually directed at external targets such as health-care professionals. It is especially important to recognise such anger for what it is and not receive it as a personal criticism. This can be difficult when the anger is sustained and is not amenable to counselling. Support from colleagues is vital in coping with this situation.

The withholding of bad news from a patient by the family may also be associated with cultural differences in emphasis on the value and nature of truth. Western Christian societies usually maintain that truth-telling is a virtue, lying is 'bad'. In medicine, there has been a steady move towards telling all patients their diagnosis. In other cultures, the concept of 'truth' may be quite different. The withholding of disturbing information may be considered more virtuous because it is considered to cause less distress. If this perspective is not recognised and respected by health-care professionals, grave difficulties in communication will arise, culminating in misunderstanding, increased anger and distress, and a collapse in the therapeutic relationship.

The problems of truth-telling are increased when the patient has a very limited understanding of the English language. Health-care professionals often resort to the use of translators to improve communication but this presents many difficulties. If the translator is a family member, he or she will be subject to the family's attitudes about breaking bad news. This will cause the translator to answer on behalf of the patient without seeming to pass on the information. Efforts to force the truth in this situation will be counter-productive. The situation may be less difficult for a professional translator who is not part of the family. However, the broad cultural constraints may be just as powerful for the professional translator as for the family. External translators may be difficult to access for urgent situations and may require payment.

Decision-making is another important area which is affected by cultural differences. Modern medical ethics stresses the importance of patient autonomy. The informed patient should be able to make his or her own decision about treatment. Quite apart from the problems of informing patients who do not speak or understand English, there can be major problems with the concept of autonomy. For extended families, the individual may not exist as an autonomous person except in so far as he or she is part of a group. Very often, there will be a decision-maker for the group, an elderly person with great status. For example, in matriarchal societies this may be a grandmother or a great aunt. They may not attend meetings with medical personnel but their influence will be very strong, even to the extent of preventing the patient from undertaking curative treatments. They must be involved in the information-giving and decision-making processes from an early stage.

Attitudes towards palliative treatments vary widely. Western medications may be viewed with mistrust. In some cultures, it may be important to bear pain stoically and minimise the expression of physical suffering. In this example, taking medications may be an admission of defeat. In other instances, medications are expected to have a one-off 'curative' effect. Thus, pain-killers are only taken once in the expectation that the pain will be cured. The taking of regular analgesics can be a very difficult concept that is only accepted by the patient after several episodes of uncontrolled pain. It is very difficult for a health-care professional to watch a patient suffer in the interim when the 'answer' seems so straight-forward. The use of complementary therapies and healers is at least as prevalent as in Western societies. The advice of these therapists may contradict the health-care professionals. If this becomes apparent, a confrontational approach to the patient and family should be avoided.

Place of death can be culturally determined. For example, many ethnic Chinese families will want dying patients to be admitted. When the death occurs in a hospital or in a hospice, the family home is less likely to be disturbed by the patient's spirit. Some families will avoid institutions completely, even when the patient is suffering from physical symptoms that might be better managed as an in-patient. If the patient is already in hospital when the family becomes aware that he or she is dying, strenuous efforts may be made to get the patient home. In other cases, the opposite happens. When patient and family have acted in seeming denial of the illness, the patient may be admitted as an 'emergency' when he or she cannot swallow. The family will usually be extremely agitated, demanding intravenous or other aggressive therapies. Many times, it will be evident that the agitation has been increased by the arrival of the extended family when the patient is dying.

When the patient dies, the expression of grief will be influenced by cultural norms. Sometimes, the emotional catharsis will seem proportional to the degree to which grief was subjugated before the death. Wailing, crying out, throwing oneself onto the body, even attempts to resuscitate the patient are some of the ways in which grief is expressed. It can be difficult accommodating these customs in an acute hospital ward or hospice in-patient unit, especially when the extended family are all present. Burial customs, such as the ritual washing and dressing of the body, must be clarified and honoured. For some, immediate burial is usual, but others may require the body to lie in state for several days. Where possible, these issues should be foreseen and planned for.

Individual Variations in Cultural Practices

Despite the broad similarities in practices and behaviours within a cultural group, there will be considerable individual variations. It is very unwise to make assumptions about the needs of a patient and family based on past experience or based on reading papers which summarise these practices. The knowledge and experience of the health-care professional should be no more than a guide. The expectations of the patient and family must be confirmed by asking them. If their needs are taken for granted and this leads to problems, an irreparable break-down in relationship may occur. Occasionally, patients and families can be made to feel very guilty because they are not conforming to the 'usual' practices that characterise their culture. An example would be assuming that a Jewish patient would only eat Kosher foods.

Variation from 'normal' cultural practices is exaggerated by the processes of assimilation and accommodation. Members of minority ethnic groups often adapt their cultural norms over time. First-generation immigrants retain a heightened awareness of their cultural origins, particularly because of the sense of loss and grief associated with leaving their native country. They often have fewer people available for support, especially if no other close relatives emigrate. Subsequent generations begin to meld with the surrounding cultures to a variable degree. However, the death of a close relative can precipitate an increased awareness of ethnic origins and even a crisis of cultural identity. In these circumstances, an even greater degree of sensitivity is needed by health-care professionals. Second-generation relatives may wear the same clothes, use many of the same mannerisms, and even have the same accent, as staff, but these similarities should not lull staff into a sense of familiarity and presumption.

Relating to Patients and Families from Other Cultures

Cross-cultural relationships, both professional and personal, must start with the health-care professional having a genuine respect for, and interest in, the other person. This does not mean that the staff member has a confident understanding of the cultural differences. Indeed, assumptions based on issues such as skin colour and ethnic status, as well as past experiences and reading, must give way to 'naive listening'. This requires the health-care professional to consider the patient and families as teachers. It also requires time, so that effective communication is established, resulting in mutual understanding. When a translator is needed, the length of an interview will be effectively doubled at least. Even when the patient and family can speak English, questions should be kept simple and answers should be straightforward. Whenever necessary, information should be written down. Drawings may also be helpful. At every point, the understanding of the patient and family should be confirmed. Opportunities for further meetings should be offered. When it is clear that a misunderstanding has occurred, always be prepared to apologise and seek clarification. Genuine efforts on the part of the health-care professional will always be rewarded with an effective and fulfilling relationship for both parties.

Bereavement Care

A terminal illness does not stop when the patient dies. The remaining family become bereaved, having lost someone who was important to them. Bereavement is a long process. There are complex and difficult emotional reactions which can be frightening, and may even threaten to overwhelm at times. Health-care professionals should know how bereavement and grief affect relatives. Many hospice services offer bereavement counselling and support. If this is not available, it is important to recognise who will benefit from support and from where this support is available. This section contains an outline of the bereavement process, a review of risk factors for an abnormal grief reaction, and some guidelines about supporting someone who is grieving. The problems of sudden or traumatic deaths not related to cancer are not dealt with.

The Bereavement Process

There is no 'normal' way to grieve. The bereavement process is a continuum which evolves according to each individual. Some common themes have been identified. However, relatives should not be required to experience their grief according to predetermined patterns. Being aware of these themes can help professionals feel more comfortable, allowing them to recognise what is happening. This helps the process of empathy.

Anticipatory Grief

When the diagnosis of a terminal illness is made, some relatives begin grieving in the weeks before the patient dies. Rarely, they share their grief with the patient. More often, they use the opportunity afforded by visiting relatives, close friends or health-care professionals to off-load feelings of sadness and impending loss. For this reason, the actual death of a terminally ill patient seems to have less of an impact than a sudden or traumatic death. Some relatives prefer to deny the seriousness of the prognosis and do not appear to experience anticipatory grief. The temptation is to encourage the person to acknowledge reality. However, denial is an important and valid coping mechanism which should not be aggressively challenged or broken down.

Relatives often try and hide their emotions for fear of upsetting the patient. They worry that exposing sadness will cause the patient to 'give up' and die more quickly. Independently, the patient may describe the same fears about sharing with the family. When this is the case, both parties can be reassured that unless there have been major problems coping with intense negative emotions in the past, the sharing of fears and sadness can be helpful. Although it is painful at the time, the catharsis can bring a sense of relief and an openness which makes the remaining time together more meaningful. This process may take place soon after the diagnosis is made or may take several weeks as people adjust to the initial shock in their own time. It cannot be expected when people have never had a trusting, sharing relationship when the patient was well.

How Do Families React when Patients Die?

It is usually obvious when cancer patients are in the last hours or days of life. The patient is often semi-conscious or comatose, unable to eat or drink, and unable to communicate. During this time, anticipatory grief may begin or intensify. Family members are often summoned to the hospital or the home. As they arrive, their grief at the obvious change in the patient's condition will trigger tears and scenes of mutual hugging and consolation. Grief reactions may be intensified by previous bereavements, as the sight of the dying patient triggers long forgotten or suppressed emotions.

Anger is the other emotion which may appear or intensify when the patient is dying. Sometimes, the anger will be directed at other members of the family. This is likely when old family conflicts are rekindled at the bedside. The anger may find expression over the patient's medical management. Relatives who have just arrived and have not been involved in the patient's care may become angry with the spouse, questioning whether everything has been done. If the patient is being cared for at home, the spouse may be so undermined that admission is required. Anger may also be directed at the doctors and nurses. Health-care professionals should not react immediately when they feel threatened but allow time for the relatives to ask all of their questions and to facilitate expression of the anger and grief. Unfortunately, junior medical staff and nurses are left to deal with these situations. Their lack of experience may compound the situation, further increasing the relatives' anger.

No matter how prepared the family members are, the actual moment of death still has an impact. When the patient stops breathing, the sudden peacefulness contrasts with the irregular, stertorous breathing that preceded it. As the realisation dawns that the irrevocable has happened, a further outpouring of strong emotions is likely. Occasionally, there may be an immediate sense of relief, particularly when the dying process has been protracted. Usually, there will be more crying; people should be encouraged to touch and kiss the body to facilitate this catharsis, if they wish. If the death has occurred unexpectedly, the emotional reactions will be more intense. Occasionally, relatives will even hurl themselves weeping or shouting on to the body. Others may rush out of the room. Any health-care professional who is present should maintain a calm demeanour, re-assuring relatives that this seemingly extreme behaviour is all right. It is often appropriate to use physical contact, such as holding a relative's hand when providing comfort, but the temptation to say something to relieve the distress, other than a brief 'I'm sorry', should be resisted. Too often, 'professional' advice becomes long-winded, uncomfortable sentences that only help the health-care professional. Sometimes, tranquillisers such as diazepam are used to help family members 'cope'. This should be avoided as it may subsequently prolong the bereavement process.

Occasionally, the moment of death is not peaceful and gentle. Although every effort may be taken to prevent such occurrences, the patient may have a haemorrhage or a convulsion, for example. The natural inclination is to rush the relatives out of the room. In fact, it may be more helpful to stand with them, encourage them to say their goodbyes and to explain what is happening – that the patient is dying – while trying to control the bleeding or the fit as calmly as possible. Relatives can usually cope if someone is with them. They should not be made to feel that they must remain but should feel free to leave the room at any time.

After relatives have vented their initial reactions to the death, the process of washing and preparing the body can begin. Cultural and religious preferences must be sought and observed. Most families leave the task to the nurses. Staff should be open to allowing family members, especially the person who has been most involved in providing physical cares, to be involved. After the body is laid out, the family can be invited to see the patient again. Observing and touching the body again can reinforce the fact that the patient has died. If a staff member is present, he or she can facilitate this by gently stroking the patient's hand from time to time and encouraging the relatives to kiss the body if they wish.

Throughout this time, children should not be forgotten. Families may want to exclude them, hoping to protect them in this way. At times, the children end up trying to protect the adults. Someone needs to focus on how they are feeling and encourage them to express themselves. Like adults, children have individual ways of coping and expressing emotions. They need honest, straightforward answers to questions and they usually want to be involved with the rest of the family. Children can be disarmingly frank about their feelings, at other times they will want to go and play as if nothing is wrong. These incongruities are part of a coping strategy that is quite natural. Parents may need encouragement to take the children to view the body after death.

After the Death

In the days that follow the death, there are many practical tasks which must be carried out. Good bereavement care concludes with the process of handing over the death certificate and the patient's belongings. In hospitals, the family often come back to a separate part of the hospital to pick up the death certificate from a stranger. No explanation is available for what is written on the certificate. The patient's belongings are often bundled together into a plastic bag. Little wonder that relatives often complain that this was one of their most traumatic experiences. In hospices, arrangements are often made for the family to come back the next day. The death certificate is reviewed with them. Advice is given about what arrangements need to made and what feelings people may experience in the next weeks. An further opportunity is given to view the body, which is very important for any family member who was not present at the time of death. With a little foresight, hospital wards can reproduce some of these personal touches, even if only to have the family return to the ward and then have a staff member accompany them to the office.

The funeral arrangements, and the funeral itself, often seem to flash by in a blur. Families busy themselves with the practical issues. At the funeral, they must maintain a level of emotional control and be able to greet, sometimes support, mourners. In other cultures, the funeral can be a time when grieving is openly encouraged. The Irish Wake and the Maori Tangi are examples of funeral celebrations which may last several days. Everyone gets to view the body lying in state. Weeping is openly encouraged. Memories of the person, good and bad, are recounted in moving and at times humorous eulogies. This process is very supportive to the extended family and greatly speeds up the emotional recovery.

After the funeral, the sense of numbness begins to subside. Feelings of intense bewilderment, loneliness, anger and sadness increase in frequency and severity. Close family will often return to their homes, leaving the spouse to cope alone. Episodes of crying will be interspersed with periods of physical inertia. Grieving relatives describe a physical sensation as if something has been wrenched from within, leaving a gaping hole inside. Other symptoms, such as loss of appetite, loss of weight, sleeplessness, restlessness, inability to concentrate, palpitations and nausea, will often drive relatives to seek medical advice. At times, they may hear the deceased person talking to them, momentarily feel the person to be physically present, or see the person walk out of a shop, for example. These reactions are all normal but they can cause the bereaved to fear that madness is setting in. Anger towards the deceased is not uncommon but can arouse considerable guilt. Reassurance may be needed that this too is normal.

As the intensity of these feelings begin to subside, people may find themselves feeling apathetic, living only from day to day, with no purpose or future. Social contacts are difficult and it is easier to stop visiting friends and family. Some people become clinically depressed. Others try to cope with their feelings by visiting friends more often. They may expect family to come around more frequently. While friends and family will excuse this need for attention initially, their patience will wear out. Then, their frustration will add to the bereaved person's emotional burden.

Recovery and reintegration takes a long time. Gradually, over a period of several months, there is an improvement in mood and energy. There are still times of sadness and yearning; the first anniversary of the death will be particularly poignant. But overall, the bereaved person will begin to establish a new identity and purpose, still utilising the memories of the dead person but integrating them into a redefined sense of self. Social contacts are re-established, new life skills are acquired, such as learning how to drive a car, and the person may embark on new directions in life.

It must be emphasised that bereavement is a normal process which most people negotiate without any need for medical or other intervention. They may benefit from some explanation about what to expect, but the support of family, friends, spiritual advisor and others, will be sufficient to see them through. The expression of grief and the mechanisms for providing support are strongly culturally determined and show wide variations (Parkes, 1997). Within these differences, however, the resilience of the human spirit still emerges through the fact that most people cope with, and reorganise, their lives.

Risk Factors for Bereavement

There are some people who do not cope with bereavement. Their lives remain severely disrupted by emotional turmoil, severe depression, or failure to redefine their personal identity. Some commit suicide, others die suddenly from natural causes. These reactions are to be distinguished from situations where bereaved relatives still continue an active life, but cling on to memories of the deceased, for example, maintaining the deceased person's bedroom unchanged as a 'shrine'. It is often possible to recognise people who are likely to have severe problems with bereavement. Several studies, notably those of Raphael (1977) and Parkes (1981) have shown that preventive bereavement counselling is effective for the high-risk bereaved.

Staff should begin assessing bereavement risks while the patient is still alive. At St Christopher's Hospice, a pictorial representation of the patient's family tree is always drawn up. The relationships between family members are illustrated and any potential problems noted. For example, the genogram may reveal that the patient's spouse has suffered multiple other bereavements in the recent past. When the patient dies, the post-death meeting with the family is used to consolidate information about how they are coping as individuals and as a unit. The relatives of patients who die at home are followed up with a phone call and then a personal visit from one of the clinical nurse specialists shortly after the funeral.

Some of the risk factors that are looked for are listed in Table 6.1.

Table 6.1   Risk factors for poor bereavement outcomes

1. The age of the patient.
2. The age of the bereaved.
3. Unexpected death (approximately 2% of cancer deaths).
4. A past history of psychiatric illness.
5. An ambivalent or dependent relationship between deceased patient and bereaved.
6. Lack of family support.
7. A history of alcohol or drug dependence.

The Age of the Patient

The death of a young patient, particularly a parent with young children, is very distressing. Aggressive anticancer treatments are often continued right up to the point when the patient dies. This gives less time for anticipatory grieving and makes the death seem more 'sudden'. Conversely, the death of an elderly person is more likely to be accepted as appropriate.

The Age of the Bereaved

While the death of an older person may be more socially acceptable, older spouses who are bereaved have greater difficulties adjusting. Elderly men are much more likely to die suddenly in the first year. Both sexes are more likely to experience increased mental and physical ill health requiring more visits to general practitioners.

Unexpected Death

About 2% of cancer deaths occur unexpectedly. Some patients die suddenly of cardiac arrest. There is also a higher incidence of events such as massive gastrointestinal bleeding, haemoptysis, pulmonary embolism and cerebral haemorrhage, which add to the distress of the death. These deaths are more likely to distress the staff as well as the relatives. This can make it more difficult for staff to recognise and address the greater needs of the bereaved.

A Past History of Psychiatric Illness

Any previous history of depression or other serious psychiatric illness can be exacerbated by bereavement. Specialist psychiatric services may have to be activated quickly if they are not already involved.

Ambivalent or Dependent Relationship Between Deceased Patient and Bereaved

Some relationships are marked by a lot of ambivalence or dependence between the partners. A long-standing 'love–hate' relationship will flare during a terminal illness when the dying patient places more demands on the partner. This causes the partner to feel angry, to hope that the patient will die quickly. When the patient does die, the partner is left feeling extremely guilty. A dependent relationship revolves around one person being 'strong', giving support and hence identity to the partner. If the dominant partner dies, the survivor may sometimes emerge dramatically, assuming new roles, almost a new personality. However, bereavement can also cause the person to feel totally bereft and helpless.

Lack of Family Support

Some bereaved partners have no family support. Worse still, the person may be isolated from family by conflicts and disputes. Disharmony will often be increased by the emotional impact of the patient's death. Grievances also focus around the contents of the deceased's will.

A History of Alcohol or Drug Dependence

Bereavement imposes a severe stress on people with alcohol and drug-dependency problems. Alcohol or drug consumption increases, adding to the difficulties that may carry over from dysfunctional relationships with the deceased. Cigarette smoking is often resumed or increased during bereavement.

Support for the Bereaved

As mentioned above, bereavement should not be considered an illness which routinely requires professionals' interventions. However, an informal visit by the family physician or community-based nursing staff who cared for the patient can be helpful. Families often use the visit to review the whole illness. They need time to talk about their current feelings, express their ongoing concerns, and ask questions. They can be given simple advice and reassurance about what to expect. The meeting will allow staff and family to bring their relationship to a close at a time when the tensions and burden of care have subsided. Whenever a bereaved spouse presents to a doctor with physical symptoms, a balanced approach is needed. Physical illnesses are more likely and symptoms should not just be ascribed to 'stress'. However, the focus of the interview should not rest on the physical problems.

For those bereaved relatives who are considered at risk of a poor bereavement outcome, several supporting options may be available, as follows:

Table 6.2   Supporting the 'at-risk' bereaved

1. Bereavement counselling services.
2. Support groups.
3. Other counselling services.
4. Specialist services.

Bereavement Counselling Services

Many hospices use trained volunteers to provide a bereavement counselling service. St Christopher's Hospice has a rigorous selection and training programme. The volunteers visit a limited number of bereaved relatives, meeting them individually on a regular basis over several weeks or months. A first visit is made 3–6 weeks after the death. The fact that the volunteer is new to the family encourages them to retell the story of what happened. This can be therapeutic in itself. On-going supervision of the volunteers is necessary because the work is emotionally demanding. Some hospital-based advisory palliative-care teams use a social worker to provide bereavement counselling.

In addition to one-to-one counselling, hospices also use larger groups to support the bereaved. Many invite relatives back to memorial services six months to one year after the patient died. The one-year anniversary of the patient's death is a very significant time. A memorial service helps to focus the grief of the bereaved. It also provides a reason for the extended family to acknowledge and share in the person's grief. Another useful method of support is small group counselling sessions which can be used to supplement or to substitute for bereavement counsellors. At St Christopher's, the bereaved relatives are told about the effects of bereavement, given advice about what to expect and offered helpful suggestions. A facilitator then guides a free discussion in which relatives share their various experiences with each other. Just hearing that other people have had the same problems is often helpful. These groups provide another opportunity to assess bereavement risk factors. Some relatives cope well initially but then begin to experience problems, particularly if their informal supports grow weary of the protracted nature of bereavement.

Support Groups

There are an increasing number of support groups established and run by bereaved people for bereaved people. They offer advice, support and sometimes counselling. They can provide a useful backup for teams that do not have a bereavement follow-up service. Some support groups serve very particular needs, such as relatives bereaved by multiple trauma or murder. Palliative care or oncology services should have current information about the groups in their local area.

Other Counselling Services

More family physicians are employing counsellors to work from the health centre. They also provide support for relatives bereaved from non-malignant as well as cancer deaths.

Specialist Services

Specialist referral to a psychiatrist or psychologist is rarely needed. They have a role in managing patients who are severely depressed, who have a recent psychiatric illness, or who express suicidal ideation and intent.

Summary

Palliative care demands that the patient and the family are treated. The cultural context is very important when assessing needs, planning care and evaluating the results of treatment. The care of families must be extended beyond the patient's death. Bereavement may be a long and difficult experience but most people manage without specialist help. Some bereaved people will develop problems. They will benefit from counselling or specialist referral.

7 – Spiritual Care and Suffering

Introduction

The modern hospice movement introduced the concept of whole person care, focusing on the spiritual as well as the physical, psychological and social needs of patients and families. Spiritual care requires a personal and a professional commitment to the patient and the family as they search for meaning in the illness. This commitment is the essence of palliative care.

Spiritual care is often mistaken as a concern for religious issues. This concern is relegated to the domain of the chaplain. The spiritual dimension is broader than the religious and involves the search for meaning and values. Many people who are facing a terminal illness become more aware of a desire to make sense of their current experience and their future. This same yearning is shared by relatives, especially the bereaved. Some people describe the experience as redefining a relationship with God; many see the spiritual as a new sense of self.

Religion has a narrower focus. It is the communal, ritualised expression of beliefs, often with strong cultural overtones. Enquiry about religious affiliation is an important part of the assessment of a terminally ill patient. This will reveal information about the frequency and importance of religious observances. Some impression about recent changes can be helpful in assessing deeper spiritual issues. The information can be used to plan how the ongoing religious needs of the patient and family can be met with sensitivity and flexibility. There is a danger that hospices which were founded on a Christian basis may impose, albeit unknowingly, specific religious practices on vulnerable, dying patients. The provision of appropriate religious care is reviewed later in this chapter.

The Role of Religious Practices in Palliative Care

Traditional religious practices are often very important for coping with death, dying, grief and loss. Even people who do not regularly attend church will seek solace in religion, perhaps harking back to childhood experiences. Each religious faith and culture has different rituals with regional and even personal variations. The care of patients from other faiths often causes concern. This concern often stems from the misconception that an expert knowledge of the culture and religion is needed before care can be attempted. Staff hold back for fear of doing or saying something which will offend. In practice, this fear is unfounded. If patients are viewed as teachers, they will advise about any special spiritual, religious or cultural needs. There have been an increasing number of books and articles about special dietary needs, rituals and customs. However, generalisations about the behaviours and attitudes of broad cultural and religious groups should not be used to predict what any individual patient will want. The key is to be sensitive and open, gently asking questions rather than allowing fear and ignorance to impede the caring relationship. Having established the needs, the staff must be committed to facilitating the patients' wishes.

Prayer is important to many patients and relatives. Some appreciate the offer of a staff member to pray with them but the offer must be made sensitively and not from religious zeal. The prayer should be short, personalised and emphasise God's support and enabling. Some hospices have prayer cards, but careful attention must be paid to the wording. Relatives may value commendatory prayers which are read when the patient dies. This can provide comfort as well as confirm that death has occurred, facilitating the start of the grieving process. Other methods can be used for patients of other faiths. Muslim patients and families may enjoy listening to readings from the Koran recorded on tape. A Buddhist patient recorded prayers and chants on a self-rewinding portable Walkman. This gave her a continuous cycle of chants which she found extremely comforting, especially at night.

Religious practices are used to mark the rites of dying and burial. Prior knowledge of these is helpful. Whenever necessary, the patient's spiritual advisor should be involved in planning for these events. This can help provide continuity of care into the bereavement period for the family. Other religious observances, such as Holy Communion, Reconciliation and even worship, should be facilitated if desired. Many hospices have a separate facility which can be used by people of different faiths for such observances. Sometimes, services will be a time of celebration, such as a wedding. These opportunities can be very moving and contribute a lot to the atmosphere of a hospice.

Spiritual Pain and Suffering

Patients often find ways of maintaining their sense of self when they are dying. Spiritual pain describes the anguish which occurs when patients cannot come to terms with their illness. It is reflected in a desperate search for meaning, expressed in questions such as 'Has my life been worth it?', 'Why is this happening to me?', or 'What have I done to deserve this?'. Another indication of spiritual pain is the expression of guilt and regret. This may concern past relationships, lost opportunities or other unfinished personal 'business'. Some people are relieved by talking about these issues, others are helped by religious rituals such as the Sacrament of Reconciliation. Occasionally, however, the desperate feelings persist and the patient becomes more and more anguished.

At times, spiritual pain may show up in other ways. Some patients, particularly the very weak, will become physically agitated. Insomnia may be another symptom as the patient lies awake, too disturbed to go to sleep. A rapid escalation in morphine dose, especially at night, can be a sign. When these signs occur, the patient will usually confirm the underlying problem when asked. However, some patients will manifest these signs but steadfastly deny or repress the underlying spiritual anguish, often denying their obvious physical deterioration as well. When the weakness of the cancer undermines the mental energy needed to maintain denial, their anguish and suffering will suddenly be released.

Suffering was defined by Cassel (1982) as 'the state of severe distress associated with events that threaten the intactness of the person'. Suffering is intensely personal in nature. The causes of suffering are perceived to be out of control, unknown, with no foreseeable end, making the patient feel helpless. The risk of personal disintegration magnifies the intensity of these perceptions.

Unfortunately, the concept of suffering has become diluted in every-day use. Phrases like 'suffering a setback' promote the idea that suffering is an unpleasant but transient reaction to an acute event. Patients who experience physical cancer pain are said to 'suffer' from pain, referring to the physical intensity of the pain. The distressing physical effects of pain, such as pain intensity and loss of sleep, remind patients of the loss of future opportunities, loss of dignity, loss of relationships and the sense of being a burden. These reminders cause spiritual pain and suffering. In some instances, a patient may be more distressed by the treatment of the pain rather than the intensity of the pain, particularly when morphine is used. Popular misconceptions about morphine abound in the minds of lay people and health-care professionals alike, misconceptions such as the fear of addiction or premature death.

Cancer pain can be considered as a metaphor for suffering; the way health-care professionals handle cancer pain can be used to understand how they respond to suffering. Cleeland et al. (1994) described the experiences of a large number of patients undergoing cancer treatments. Many patients reported uncontrolled pain despite the high levels of knowledge which physicians had about pain control. Most patients received inadequate pain treatments. Even more worrying were the non-medical factors which appeared to influence pain management. For example, young women, the elderly and patients from ethnic minorities were more likely to have uncontrolled pain. As mentioned in Chapter 1, these problems are often attributed to the emergence of high-technology treatments and investigations which have led doctors to focus on the cancer rather than the patient. A critical examination of medical history reveals that doctors have always found the care of the dying to be difficult.

Why Do Health-Care Professionals Have Difficulty Managing Suffering?

There are many factors which make it difficult for health-care professionals to recognise and deal with suffering. Health-care professionals, especially physicians, tend to come from higher socio-economic groups. They will probably only have a limited personal experience of suffering. Younger staff are unlikely to have experienced a major physical illness; their parents and even their grandparents will often still be alive. A first-hand experience of illness is not a prerequisite for working in the caring professions, indeed major problems will occur if practice is based on past personal experience. However, if handled correctly, personal experience can improve empathy when balanced with professional detachment and self-awareness. Without this experience, empathy towards the suffering of others must be actively taught.

Health-care professionals are also people. Most people fear death. This fear operates at a subconscious level, making people intolerant of situations which are associated with death and dying. Solomon et al. (1995) showed that subjects exposed to videos illustrating death distanced themselves from people who had different cultural norms and expectations. This same reaction occurs when staff are confronted with suffering. One method of distancing from a threatening situation is to relabel the problem so that it is no longer perceived as a problem. Relabelling is often seen with cancer patients. Wilkes (1984) found that physicians consistently under-reported pain and over-reported patient anxiety. By redefining pain as anxiety, the patient becomes the 'problem' not the pain or the physician's lack of knowledge about pain control.

Professional training can increase the problems of dealing with suffering. Medicine is taught as a science. Scientific methods include dispassionate observation of measurable facts which are then arranged into patterns. Diseases are taught as discrete entities with specific clinical findings. The frequent embellishments which patients add during history-taking are often disregarded, even though they contain powerful messages about patients' fears. Most clinical teaching occurs in acute hospitals where the emphasis is on diagnosis and cure. Little teaching is provided about the care of the whole person or the nature of suffering. Occasionally, communication skills are taught but information about pain control is minimal. Medical students are not allowed to say 'I don't know'. This 'training' prevents doctors from acknowledging deficits in knowledge which then encourages avoidance strategies such as walking past the room of a dying person on a ward round. The training of nurses is more likely to include teaching about palliative care. However, this knowledge will be undermined if doctors are not able to support requests from nurses for better pain control of their patients.

After qualification, staff find that pressure of work undoes any training in communication skills. Verbal and non-verbal methods are used to minimise the stress of patient contacts. Examples include the use of questions which are not open-ended, ignoring patient cues to talk about distressing issues and using body language which indicates impatience to end the interview. These strategies are reinforced by the role models of senior colleagues. The fact that cancer patients want to please health-care professionals only makes these problems worse.

In summary, there are many personal and professional reasons why staff find it difficult to recognise and deal with suffering. Most people want to avoid distressing situations, particularly if they lack the knowledge or skills to handle these situations. Avoidance techniques such as relabelling are reinforced by professional training. The next section outlines how suffering can be managed.

The Management of Suffering

The management of suffering requires a team approach. Each member of the team must recognise and value the contribution and skills of the others. The information which doctors gain, for example, is heavily influenced by patients wanting to say things which do not upset them. Patients will often give a different view to other health-care professionals. Combining the various perspectives ensures that each member of the team will have a more complete picture of the problems.

Although team members have different professional skills which can be bought to bear, the most important response to someone who is suffering is a caring human presence. Staying with the patient, not flinching or hurrying away from the anguish, will help to counter the feelings of isolation and abandonment felt by the terminally ill. The need of the carer to console may be overwhelming at times but it is important to be comfortable in sitting, listening to the struggle, the pain, the unanswerable questions. People who are suffering need to be understood, to have their experiences confirmed. Active listening is hard work. It requires time, patience and commitment, alongside a non-judgemental approach that accepts whatever the patient wants to say, whatever way he or she wants to say it.

Suffering is focused on the future. Some questions may help to elicit the patient's fears for the future, for example 'What is the worst thing that you imagine is going to happen to you?' This may provoke dramatic and vivid images. Patients may describe the cancer as rotting away inside the body or may be concerned that the abdomen will rupture from ascites. When these perceptions have little basis in medical fact, a careful and simple explanation may bring enormous relief. Uncontrolled physical symptoms will frighten patients, making them worry about dying in agony. This emphasises the need to relieve symptoms and assure patients that other options are available if needed in the future.

The family may help to shed light on a patient's suffering. However, relatives often load their own distress into their perceptions of the patient. Consequently, their views must be interpreted cautiously. The character of the patient prior to the illness and the past experiences with other relatives who have died of cancer are two examples of information which may help put the patient's suffering into context. Sometimes, a joint meeting with the patient and family can be helpful. Patients often worry about becoming a burden. They seldom express these fears to the carers, and become increasingly anguished for the relatives who in turn are affected by the patients' distress. Openly addressing these worries can be very liberating.

Patient support groups can be an important resource. People who come together with similar experiences can quickly develop an atmosphere of understanding and mutual support. Practical solutions to problems will often be shared. The heart-felt sense of 'being in it together' can have a powerful therapeutic effect, overcoming helplessness and isolation. While some groups have operated successfully without a facilitator, it is often helpful to have a trained professional present.

Suffering is often associated with intense anger. Patients may have problems expressing their rage about the illness. The family may find themselves subjected to angry outbursts, the more frightening if the patient normally had a placid nature. The distress of the family will be increased by the patient's maintaining an easy-going 'front' with visitors or health-care professionals. Staff can help the family by helping patients develop an alternative focus for their anger. Patients can often be encouraged to express their anger more appropriately. For example, giving a patient permission to be angry with God may help, especially when previous religious upbringing would regard this as blasphemy.

Spiritual care is primarily about staying alongside patients who have un-answerable questions, who struggle to make sense of an illness without meaning. The desire to say something helpful can be overwhelming but usually only results in a non-verbal message that the listener cannot handle the distress. Most patients are not actually looking for an answer. They know that there is no explanation but there is a need to express the conflict or distress. Just talking about the issues can be therapeutic. Verbalising the deep-seated fears can some-times make the issues more concrete, less frightening, and more controllable.

This approach to spiritual care can cause major problems for some people who work in palliative care. They see it as too passive. Patients should be able to find meaning in the illness, meaning which is expressed as an acceptance of dying. The 'good death' is characterised by a calm acquiescence, the resolution of unfinished business and a relaxed physical demeanour. However, studies have shown that only a small proportion of patients want to die in this way. Most want to die in 'ordinary life', struggling to maintain a familiar routine until the end (Kastenbaum, 1988). If the health-care professionals' goal is to make patients accept their illness, there is grave risk that patients' suffering will be made worse.

What if Suffering is not Relieved?

Listening to patients' anguish, correcting misinformation, controlling symptoms and addressing other unmet needs usually restores their sense of control. This does not mean that feelings of sadness, frustration, anger, uncertainty and anxiety do not recur from time to time. The intensity of these feelings will be less and there is no longer the same sense of impending personal disintegration. However, a few patients remain deeply anguished and their suffering will con-tinue unabated.

When suffering is not relieved, it is important to ask for advice from a specialist palliative-care service. There is no place for professional pride when the spiritual well-being of a patient is at stake. Sometimes, a psychiatric review will be helpful to exclude a diagnosis of agitated depression. A past history of depression or a family history of depression may be helpful pointers. A trial of antidepressants may be warranted. Unfortunately, many psychiatrists lack experience in assessing terminally ill patients. Also, psychiatric services are increasingly stretched by increasing workload and lack of resources.

If the options have been exhausted, the value of a team approach becomes apparent. Staff can support each other and share the task of spending time with the patient. This prevents any one staff member from being overwhelmed and taking action which threatens the autonomy of the patient, such as using heavy sedation. Family members must be supported as well. They will be even more affected by the helplessness of only being able to watch the patient's distress.

Rarely, some cancer patients become extremely distressed when they are dying. When they become too weak to get out of bed, they also lose the mental energy needed to maintain the denial or control the anguish. Physicians often fail to recognise the significance of the extreme agitation. Urgent treatment is required. Sedation will usually be necessary with subcutaneous injections of midazolam. The major tranquillisers, such as chlorpromazine or methotri-meprazine, can also be given parenterally. Sometimes, they have a paradoxical effect, making the agitation worse. Diazepam has a limited role because of difficulties with administration: the oral route is rarely available and the rectal route is a problem when the patient is unsettled. Some patients do not respond or become tolerant to the effect of these drugs. High doses of phenobarbitone need to be considered, 200 mg every 15 minutes until the patient is settled. A minimum maintenance dose of 200 mg will be needed four hourly.

A decision to use sedation should not be devolved to the family, although they must be involved in the discussions. Most relatives experience an initial sense of relief when the patient is settled. However, feelings of guilt may then emerge and need to be addressed. Sometimes, the reason for using sedatives has to be revisited because the relatives want the patient to be 'woken up' and to be normal again. A careful explanation of the problems will be needed because a decrease in the dose of the sedatives is rarely possible. It will cause extreme agitation to recur.

Supporters of euthanasia argue that 'suffering' patients should be given a lethal injection. This is viewed as a humane alternative to sedation. In practice, these patients rarely ask for euthanasia. Even when a patient does ask, the request is more often a cry for help and understanding. If euthanasia were more available, the request is likely to be taken at face value. There are even more serious consequences of legalising euthanasia which are reviewed in Chapter 11 on ethical issues in palliative care. It is significant that in Holland, where there is a liberal euthanasia policy, there is are hardly any specialist palliative-care services. The response to suffering is not euthanasia but better training and greater availability of palliative care.

Improving the Management of Suffering

Teaching about suffering, symptom control and palliative care should be available at all stages of training for health-care professionals. Didactic teaching is the simplest option but can only convey a limited view. Good role models are also needed in teaching hospitals. This can be provided by specialist advisory palliative-care teams or hospital-based palliative-care units.

Training should also address the personal and professional issues which prevent health-care professionals from recognising and treating suffering. Issues such as racism and sexual discrimination should be reviewed. Students should be exposed to other cultures and other models of care such as hospices. Speakers from patient groups, ethnic minorities and religious communities can be used to expand awareness. Every opportunity should be taken to encourage multi-professional teaching. This can be enhanced by using assignments which require group working for results, countering the usual emphasis on personal learning and achievement. Teaching of communication skills must be increased.

Conclusion

The suffering patient provides a challenge that demands a high level of personal as well as professional commitment. Helping someone regain control of the future is very rewarding and more than compensates for the cost. Health-care professionals must collaborate to achieve this. For the patient, relief from fear and uncontrolled symptoms will allow the following months to become a positive chance to mend or strengthen relationships, grasp new opportunities and achieve a greater sense of positive self-awareness. However, occasionally it is not possible to relieve suffering. When this happens, staff need to continue supporting the patient, but they will also need support for each other and for the family.

8 – Teamwork and Palliative Care

Introduction

Throughout this book, the importance of inter-disciplinary teamwork has been emphasised as a fundamental principle of palliative care. There are many examples of inter-professional working in other areas of health care, for example, gerontology and paediatrics. In palliative care, the degree of role overlap between disciplines, coupled with the inherent stresses of working with the terminally ill, create particular difficulties. This chapter focuses on how teamworking can be achieved. The definition of a team is explored, followed by a review of the roles played by team members. Selection of team members is examined and the chapter concludes with an analysis of the strategies needed to maintain team cohesion.

What is Teamwork?

Many people think of a team as a collection of individuals with a common geographic base, for example, the team that works on a particular ward or in a specific department. However, a team is a functional dynamic entity which is defined by a task or tasks that can only be accomplished if the team members work together. It is the collaborative effort in pursuit of common goals that characterises teamwork. The members of a team need to agree upon, and be committed to, a common set of tasks and goals. In palliative care, the overall goal is to address the needs of the patients and families. Advisory palliative-care services may also have the secondary goal of supporting the other staff directly involved in the care of patients and families.

Although the main goal of a palliative-care team relates to patients and families in general, each clinical situation will bring forth specific tasks that apply to each individual case. In some instances, the needs of a particular patient or family member will exceed the aggregate abilities and experience of the team members. In these instances, the 'team' will need to be expanded to include other health-care professionals or appropriate specialists if the goal is to be achieved. This broad approach to teamwork helps to maintain the focus on the task, rather than the individual members. It reinforces the importance of a multi-disciplinary approach. Medical problems cannot become the sole priority, as is characteristic of the traditional medical model.

111

Setting Limits

Specific limits may need to be built into team objectives. Palliative-care teams sometimes restrict the type of patients that are accepted for care. For example, palliative-care services are often expert at managing pain problems. This may lead to referral of patients with chronic benign non-malignant pain, particularly if there is no pain clinic. However, this group of patients has quite different problems and needs from terminally ill patients. Most teams do not accept these patients. Several teams restrict their services to terminally ill cancer patients because they are not confident in managing the problems associated with the variety of progressive non-malignant diseases. Teams working in in-patient hospice units may restrict referrals to patients with a relatively short prognosis, usually less than one month.

The Role of Team Members

Palliative-care teams are usually made up of members from several disciplines: nurses, doctors, social workers, secretarial staff and clergy. Some community-based 'teams' may only comprise two or three nurses, but they are not as effective operating in isolation from other professionals. If other disciplines are not represented, at least there should be an informal network of colleagues for additional advice and support. Some teams also include physiotherapists, occupational therapists and pharmacists. Volunteers, bereavement counsellors and health visitors also work as an integral part of some teams. Support staff, such as managers, domestic cleaners and cooks are important in the in-patient setting.

With so many disciplines potentially working together, each member of a team should have a role which is clearly understood. Defining a role begins with a practical job description. This is essential when selecting team members. Applicants must know what the job entails and the interviewers must have a basis for assessing their suitability. Once staff are in post, a realistic under-standing of each person's role will make for greater team effectiveness and harmony. Regular appraisal will compare the individual's role with the job description, thereby identifying strengths and weaknesses, opportunities for professional development, and clarification of specific goals for the next year.

The tasks, responsibilities and skills required for a palliative-care team are wide ranging. The following profiles are not prescriptive or complete. They serve to illustrate the breadth of multi-skilling that is characteristic of this speciality.

Nurses

Nurses constitute the greater proportion of professional care-givers within palliative care. Hospice in-patient units deliberately over-staff wards to enable sufficient time for patient and family care. Staffing levels may be up to one-third more than comparably-sized acute hospital wards. This enables the high standards of nursing care which are demanded in hospices to be met. The role of nurses has been extended beyond the performance of physical cares. The close physical contact with terminally ill patients makes nurses very aware of symptom control and emotional needs. With adequate training, nurses are capable of assessing these needs, initiating psychological support and adjusting treatment regimens. A range of doses for morphine is often prescribed in hospices so that nurses can use their clinical judgement to increase the dose if necessary. Similarly, a range of other drugs such as sedatives, anti-emetics and anti-cholinergics are prescribed on the 'prn' sheet so that nurses can initiate these treatments if a patient deteriorates, without having to wait for a doctor to assess the patient. Nurses have a vital role in maintaining contact with relatives: listening to their concerns, answering questions, assessing how the individual members are coping and then liaising with other team members. The training of palliative-care nurses has been recognised by the introduction of degree and diploma courses offered by academic nursing centres.

Although working in a hospice provides experience in symptom management and emotional care, it does not prepare for the major stresses associated with applying this experience in an advisory role. Community and hospital-based advisory teams need to use nurse specialists. They have an even higher degree of knowledge and expertise. This is needed to evoke respect from the nursing and medical staff who are seeking advice. Many community-based teams also require that applicants have district nurse or health visitor qualifications. Teaching and education are an important part of the nurse specialist's role. These functions can provide an enjoyable and stimulating balance to the more demanding advisory role. Practical 'hands-on' care is only rarely carried out, usually as an adjunct to the teaching.

The pathways of responsibility and accountability for nurse specialists need to be carefully defined. Acute hospital services and government-funded community teams are often made responsible to senior nurses or administrators who are physically remote from the team. They may be very supportive if they have an adequate understanding of palliative care and a strong commitment to the success of the team. If support is not forthcoming at this level, severe distress occurs and may result in the collapse of the service. Diffusion of accountability, when different nurses on a team have different supervisors, will also produce significant tensions.

Doctors

Palliative-care teams usually have at least one doctor. Some home-care teams work without a doctor but this places more stress on the non-medical team members when they have to advise on medical issues. Hospital-based advisory teams without a doctor find it difficult to establish credibility within the hospital, particularly with the medical staff. Doctors come to palliative care from a wide variety of backgrounds including oncology, radiotherapy, psychiatry, clinical pharmacology, anaesthetics, general medicine, surgery and general practice. As with nurse specialists, the credibility of the doctor will depend on being able to control difficult palliative-care problems. Training is necessary to achieve this.

Recently, training in palliative-care medicine has been officially recognised in the United Kingdom and Australasia. Postgraduate qualifications are now available. The professional colleges in several countries have accepted, or are working towards, specialty training in palliative care. If a doctor has not been trained in palliative medicine, then the prior training of the doctor may limit how a palliative-care team functions. An anaesthetist with an interest in nerve blocks, for example, causes the team to function more like a pain-management service with an emphasis on interventional strategies. Other symptoms or psycho-social needs would then be ignored or treated less well. A doctor who has trained in oncology or radiotherapy may get referrals from these specialities but other doctors will be worried that their patients may be 'taken over'.

Doctors have an important role in assessing and prescribing treatment for symptom control problems. Nurses can become very proficient, even to the extent of providing advice about medication changes for many problems. However, there are situations which require a more detailed medical history and examination before the cause of the symptom or the best treatment can be established. Many patients and families need the reassurance of talking to a doctor about the diagnosis or treatment. The doctor may be more aware of the rarer manifestations of cancer, as well as the management of non-malignant conditions, such as heart-failure, for example. Some cancer patients may have other illnesses which necessitate using conventional palliative-care strategies in a different way. For example, renal impairment will cause delays with morphine clearance. A doctor is more likely to know how to adapt to these situations using the first principles of pharmacology.

In the hospice setting, the doctor will be responsible for the medical super-vision of in-patients. Doctors working on advisory teams in the community or in hospital do not have direct responsibility for patient care. This responsibility remains with the general practitioner or the hospital consultant. It can be extremely difficult for a doctor to relinquish this role. Having to negotiate every investigation or change in medication can be disheartening and humiliating, especially if advice is ignored and patient care suffers. Whereas general practi-tioners and ward-based medical teams will often respond to the advice of nurse specialists on advisory teams, there are times when the doctor needs to lend authority to the situation. More stress will be imposed on the team if the doctor avoids this responsibility. This role needs to be exercised to avoid undermining the status of the nurse specialist or damaging relationships within the team.

Doctors have a role in supporting the other members of the team, especially providing back-up information and advice to nurse specialists on advisory teams. This role may be confused with the issue of professional control, leading to problems within the team. Doctors may have difficulty working alongside other disciplines, preferring to be the leader of the team. The supportive role of the doctor depends on continuity of medical input, which can become an issue if the doctor is only employed part-time. Attendance at multi-disciplinary meet-ings can be undermined if the doctor has a heavy case load elsewhere. The resultant stress on the team members can be considerable and may cause the team to collapse (Herxheimer et al., 1985).

Doctors working in palliative medicine often have a teaching role. Opportun-ities to teach medical students, junior doctors and general practitioners are vital to promote better palliative care. Where possible, other members of the team should be involved to illustrate the multidisciplinary approach. Doctors can also teach other members of other disciplines. For example, teaching for district nurses can improve the care of patients in the community by giving them more confidence when discussing treatment changes with the general practitioners. The promotion of research and publication is an important adjunct to the teaching role in the medical school and teaching hospitals.

Despite the specific contributions that a doctor can make, there is considerable potential for role overlap, especially with nurses. This can lead to conflict and frustration for both disciplines. Whenever role conflict is perceived, time should be spent discussing and resolving the problem. Sometimes, role overlap will be imposed inappropriately. For example, if a hospice unit has inadequate medical cover, the nurses may find themselves having to shoulder too much responsibility, which then causes anxiety and role overload. If there is no option for increasing the hours which the doctor works or the number of doctors, the nurses may not openly discuss the problem for fear of losing what little doctoring is available.

Social Workers

The traditional roles of social workers include helping families with social, emotional or practical problems. This means that social work has an important complementary role in palliative care. Social workers may have a practical role with issues such as co-ordination of discharge planning, as well as identifying appropriate financial and other welfare resources. Unfortunately, many team members perceive these as the only functions that a social worker can contribute. Many teams do not include a social worker. Instead, they rely on liaising with social workers employed by other agencies who may not be as familiar or confident with these needs. Suitable training is needed to recognise and deal with some of the particular needs of the terminally ill.

The social worker can assess how physical, emotional and social factors combine to influence the patient and family. This helps remind other team members that every patient is part of a social system which influences the patient's behaviour and perception of the illness. The social worker can also provide a greater understanding of the possible strengths and resources possessed by families. Social workers can help patients and families explore relationships, especially with children, and weaken the barriers caused by strong emotions such as anger, guilt, sadness and regret. Joint interviews by the social worker and nurse or doctor will increase the effectiveness of the interviews.

The social worker often has a role as advocate between patients, families and staff. The advocacy role may be facilitated by the perceived non-medical status of social work. This perception by patients and families can make it easier to ask important questions which they have not felt able to ask of the doctors and nurses. These questions can then be directed to the appropriate staff members.

Social workers are often involved with bereavement care. The provision of bereavement follow-up is sometimes carried out by the social worker. Relatives who are thought to be at risk of a difficult bereavement may be seen individually or in groups. Some hospice bereavement services use trained volunteers. The social worker then provides training and supervision.

In the same way that the social worker often has a more holistic view of the patient and family, he or she is often in a better position to monitor how the other disciplines work as a team. The social worker can monitor feelings within the team and then facilitate better team working. However, because counselling skills and a holistic approach to caring are not the sole prerogative of social work, the social worker may feel threatened by role overlap with the doctors and nurses. Attention is needed to prevent this potential overlap from causing conflict which undermines team working.

Spiritual Advisors

Palliative care stresses the importance of the spiritual dimension. This means that spiritual advisors have an integral role in supporting patients facing a terminal illness, although not all patients will want direct involvement. The distinction between religious and spiritual care is made in Chapter 7 which highlighted some of the religious practices which are pertinent to palliative care. Some hospices have chaplains who minister to the religious and spiritual needs of patients and families. Other hospices liaise with the patient's usual spiritual advisor. Hospital-based teams often make use of hospital chaplaincy services. Palliative-care services must also build relationships with non-Christian spiritual advisors, particularly for the significant minority ethnic groups who are present in the catchment area. These advisors can provide valuable information about the religious needs and observances that are associated with death and dying in all cultures. Better awareness will also encourage referral when a patient is admitted to the hospice. Written information, including contact telephone numbers, should be available to staff.

Some chaplains who have not trained in palliative care will have difficulty dealing with dying patients and their families. This can limit their involvement to administering the basic religious requirements such the Sacrament of the Sick, or reading prayers for the dying. Many chaplains enjoy counselling patients and families, and their role will naturally extend to the care of relatives into the bereavement period. The counselling role may overlap with other members of the team and cause conflict.

There are many other roles which may be performed by spiritual advisors, depending on their skills and interests. Chaplains may play an active part in teaching medical, nursing, social work and other students. As with social work, spiritual advisors may fulfil a patient advocate role. They may also play an important role in supporting the team. He or she may be used as a confidant by team members, or as someone who facilitates the examination and resolution of team conflict.

Volunteers

Volunteers have become a vital part of the modern hospice movement. Hospices rely heavily on their input, particularly those hospices which are charities. The use of volunteers requires careful organisation and support, usually by a volunteer co-ordinator. Recruitment of volunteers is usually not difficult but rigorous selection and training is essential. Attention must also be paid to the legal and insurance implications of using volunteers.

There are several roles which are fulfilled by volunteers. Although the tasks may be very practical, the associated contact with patients and families can be important. For example, volunteer drivers may provide transport for patients to clinics and day-care facilities. During the journey, the patient will often confide fears and anxieties. Secretarial and administrative functions may be undertaken by volunteers, particularly retired civil servants, accountants and other professionals. Volunteers also play a vital role in organising and carrying out fundraising activities. Bereavement follow-up can be provided by volunteers, but they need careful training and supervision.

There is an increasing trend to use volunteers for patient and family care. They can stay with patients at home, giving relatives the opportunity for a break. Patients without family can be befriended by a volunteer if they do not want to feel so isolated by the illness. Performing tasks such as gardening and shopping can also be helpful. Volunteers have a major role in day hospices. They help with activities, preparing meals and socialising with patients.

The use of volunteers may seem to result in cost savings. However, they should never be used with the primary intention of saving money. This is particularly true for tasks which require a full-time commitment. Another problem which must be constantly addressed is the potential for conflict between volunteers and paid staff. Professionals may look down on volunteers, thereby undervaluing their contribution. This can be minimised by proper training of paid and volunteer staff. These issues emphasise the importance of a volunteer services co-ordinator.

Administration

In most countries, hospice services rely heavily on charitable sources of funding. Very few are totally or even majority funded from government. Palliative care is a time-intensive, and therefore labour-intensive, speciality. All but the smallest services need personnel for fundraising and administrative functions. These functions will not be discussed further in this book. Clear lines of management are needed to ensure the smooth running of the hospice and minimal disruption to clinical services. A key principle of palliative care is that clinical staff should have easy and comfortable relationships with the administrative staff.

Recruitment of Team Members

The process of recruiting to a palliative-care service is very important. It is a demanding speciality which cannot be undertaken lightly. A wrong appointment can disrupt a team and will seriously affect the person who is appointed. The formal interview is a crucial time for assessing potential applicants. A picture of the whole person must be built up, based on an assessment of past work experience and achievements, personality, interpersonal skills and coping strategies. Enquiry should be made about past and current stressful events, particularly the death of someone close. The aim is to understand how the applicant has handled major losses, which may indicate how the person will respond to the stresses of palliative care. Many services exclude people who have had a recent bereavement or other significant loss. Other character traits such as stability, ability to relate well and to handle pressure, should be evaluated. Any signs of emotional immaturity, such as poor self-control, dependence or show-off tendencies will indicate that the person is not suitable.

Team Meetings

Effective team working requires close collaboration. Team meetings are often needed to formalise this. Regular clinical meetings are used as a forum for discussing patients' and families' problems, then devising treatment strategies. The traditional medical model requires the doctor to be the team leader of these meetings. However, this model has important consequences for the dynamics of meetings and can limit the effectiveness of the team. The biggest problem is that 'leader' is often synonymous with 'decision-maker'. The doctor may tend to make decisions on a unilateral basis, usually focusing on medical problems. Non-medical staff often feel compelled to stay quiet when they disagree. They find it difficult to raise non-medical issues. This undermines their confidence, and limits their effectiveness and contributions. The commitment of team members to action decisions made by the doctor will be weaker. Difficulties will also arise if the doctor is frequently unavailable between meetings. For advisory teams, the doctor-lead model will make nurse specialists less confident about making urgent clinical decisions at the patient's bedside.

If teams want to develop beyond the traditional model, determination is required to break down conventional, status-determined patterns of thinking and inter-relating. Conscious efforts must be made to affirm and value the observations and opinions of all team members. This means overcoming another common trait within the health professions: not giving due praise because a professional is 'only doing a job'. Senior team members, particularly the doctor, should be sure that they do not cut short information from other team members. The aim should be to encourage a broad-ranging discussion, building up a variety of strategies based on collective experience rather than opting for the 'right' way. This model is also better suited to dealing with non-medical problems.

Dealing with Team Conflict

Conflict is inevitable in any team. Palliative care is a potentially stressful speciality, given the emotional load inherent in the suffering experienced by patients and families. Palliative-care teams need mechanisms and strategies for managing stress and conflict. Review meetings are often held regularly, remaining distinct from the daily or weekly clinical meetings. A few teams make use of an 'objective' facilitator for review meetings – someone who is not normally part of the team.

Team reviews should be used for sharing professional anxieties and stresses. For reviews to be useful, team members should become familiar with the causes and manifestations of stress within themselves and their colleagues (Vachon, 1987). Stress can lead to physical symptoms, such as fatigue, weight change and sleep disturbance. The psychological effects include anger, irritability and frustration. All of these will generate conflicts in the team as well as in the individual's private life. If stress is not recognised or dealt with, the team member will lose confidence, will experience difficulty in making or implementing decisions, and eventually will be incapable of performing his/her job. For hospice-based teams, the problems often centre difficult symptom control or psycho-social issues. Reflecting back on 'difficult' deaths can analyse what contributed to the stresses and can define alternative strategies to prevent similar problems from recurring. Advisory palliative-care teams in hospitals face these same challenges but they also have less direct control over treatments. They need to use review sessions as a way of venting frustrations about people outside the team: the 'unco-operative' doctors, 'unfeeling' nurses, etc who may contribute to inadequate clinical outcomes.

Personality and professional conflicts within the team are often more difficult to deal with. The usual tendency is to suppress disagreement and conflict. This leads to 'chronic niceness', with each team member hiding ill-feelings, pretending outwardly that nothing is wrong. While this may maintain the functional integrity of the team in the short-term, the pressures on the facade will grow, especially if there are other stresses on the team. Eventually, the mental energy needed to maintain an illusion of team cohesion will impair from the team's clinical performance. Another short-lived way of easing tension is for team members to discuss a problem with others on the team but not with the person who is perceived to be the cause of the conflict. In the long term, this causes factions and further disruption. Some people cope by talking to family and friends after work, but if the underlying cause is not resolved, this strategy will disrupt these relationships.

Overcoming 'chronic niceness' is very difficult. It is vital to build up an atmosphere of trust and mutual respect, especially by encouraging team members' skills and strengths. This requires sharing personal successes and achievements as a team, allowing others to give due praise. Affirmation has to be realistic and not paternalistic. It can take several months before team members feel safe enough with each other to explore disagreements, to overcome the feeling that criticism is a personal attack. In a supportive atmosphere, constructive solutions can be explored to professional and personal conflicts. It may be necessary to use an outside facilitator if conflicts are very deep-seated or seemingly insoluble.

Team dynamics are often improved by social gatherings. Pub lunches, picnics, theatre visits and other outings are relaxing and therapeutic. They also stop reviews from becoming too sombre and introspective. Team members, particularly new ones, establish relationships with each other more readily.

Training Team Members

Staff stress is always increased if they lack the knowledge and skills for addressing patients' and families' needs. Training is a powerful way of reducing stress by making the job more rewarding. There is a sense of personal and professional growth, coupled with the satisfaction of providing a better service. Team members should support one another by encouraging study leave and training opportunities. Staff appraisals help to formalise this process and allow the administration to confirm a commitment to training.

A way of improving clinical knowledge is for team members to research problems which arise in practice, and then present a short summary to the team. This can improve self-confidence and further break down the traditional doctor-centred model of team working. Courses and seminars are another valuable way to increase knowledge. They also help to overcome any sense of isolation for palliative-care services that are small and isolated. There are many conferences on palliative care. An increasing number are organised by the professional colleges and academies. However, the acquisition of new skills requires more than the acquisition of knowledge. Skills need to be developed and refined in a supervised environment. For staff who are new to palliative care, practical skills can be gained by working in a hospice. Counselling and teaching skills can often be improved in workshops. The traditional model of doctor teaching doctor, nurse teaching nurse and social worker teaching social worker has been broken down. This has further strengthened the team approach.

Summary

The complex problems of terminally ill patients and their families cannot be resolved by any one individual or profession. Palliative-care services are based on professionals and volunteers working in teams. The team is defined by task or tasks which can only be fulfilled by the collaborative efforts of the members, not by its geographic location or composition. In palliative care, there is often overlap in the roles of the team members. Careful selection and training is needed to help new team members cope with this. Effective teams also need to work consciously at moving beyond the traditional medical-centred model of team-working in health care. Explicit mechanisms are also needed to deal with stress and conflict. The next chapter reviews the practical aspects of palliative-care teams working in different environments, including home care, in-patient hospice units and hospitals.

9 – Delivering Palliative Care in Different Settings

Introduction

The previous chapters have outlined strategies and techniques for managing the variety of physical, emotional, social and spiritual problems associated with advanced cancer. The setting in which patients and families are cared for has an important influence on how these strategies are implemented. Palliative care was first developed in the in-patient hospice setting. However, the principles of palliative care were quickly adapted to the care of terminally ill patients at home. Although the number of in-patient units has grown rapidly, the even greater emphasis on home care properly reflects the fact that cancer patients spend most of the last six months of life at home.

Another important setting of care is acute hospitals. Although there are more hospices, most cancer patients die in hospital. Multiple admissions and out-patient visits to hospitals are common in the last year of life. Many patients are treated by specialised cancer treatment services. As more anti-cancer treatments become available, and as more people become aware of these options, the use of these services is increasing. For other patients, hospital care is provided by general medical and surgical services. All of these factors have prompted different ways of bringing palliative care into the acute-care setting. With the expanding population of the very elderly, the provision of good palliative care in residential and nursing homes is receiving more attention.

The practice of palliative care has to be adapted to suit the different opportunities, constraints and needs which arise in different environments. This chapter reviews these adaptations, starting with the strategies needed to promote home care. The characteristics of in-patient hospices are then outlined, followed by consideration of approaches which have been used to improve care in hospitals and other institutions. Special attention is given to the practice of palliative care within the acute oncology setting.

Palliative Care at Home

Most cancer patients prefer to be at home. Those patients who can express a choice will say that they want to die at home. However, only a minority of these patients will actually achieve their choice. This testifies to the major difficulties that confront cancer patients and their families at home. Patients who are physically well enough and who want to stay at home will usually have little initial difficulty in doing so. They will maintain a semblance of normal activity and will participate in the control of significant emotional and other tensions. However, as the physical effects of cancer take hold, patients become weaker, begin to experience more frequent and severe symptoms, and become less able to control their own or other people's fears and anxieties. While some patients become so physically exhausted that they accept what is happening, others become so frightened that their fear overrides any desire to stay at home.

For the family, there are several factors which undermine their ability to care for a patient at home. The sense of impending loss increases as the patient deteriorates. Carers struggle to control their own emotions as they try to protect the patient. On to this emotional background is loaded the even greater distress of helplessness. Family carers often try to reassure and console patients but feel that these attempts are ineffective. The few things that lay people are normally confident to do, such as making meals, become progressively less effective and then become burdensome to the patient. Another factor is the overwhelming sense of responsibility felt by the carers. They often believe that only health-care professionals can provide adequate care, particularly when the patient is experiencing symptoms or is dying. Relatives live in fear of doing something that will make the patient's suffering worse, leaving a burden of guilt for the rest of their lives. All of these psychological factors are exacerbated by the fatigue of providing physical care. It is little wonder that so few patients die at home.

With careful planning and support, patients and families can overcome many of the barriers to care in the home. One of the most satisfying aspects of home care is hearing relatives proudly say after the patient has died at home 'We never thought that we could have done that'. The sense of achievement often goes some way to helping with the sense of loss. That is not to say that the aim of home care is to make all people die at home; this will create even more distress and guilt for those families who cannot care for the patient at home. Even for these families, it should be possible to give them a greater sense of control and security while the patient is at home, and later to ameliorate any sense of guilt that they may experience when the patient eventually dies in hospital.

Strategies for Promoting Palliative Care at Home

The basis of promoting palliative care at home is the empowerment of patients and their carers, giving them the confidence needed to overcome uncertainty and fear. The strategies needed to empower families and patients are listed in Table 9.1.

Many of these strategies can and should be implemented as early as practicable in the course of the illness.

Maintaining Regular Contact

Regular visits to the home can reduce the anxiety of home care. The frequency of the visits should be tailored to the disease progression and the needs of the patient and family. When the patient first presents with symptoms of advanced cancer, frequent visits may be needed to assess the problems and establish control. If the situation stabilises, occasional monthly or fortnightly contacts, often by telephone, may be all that is necessary. Some health-care professionals find it hard to make contact if there is nothing practical to be done. However, most patients and families feel reassured. Some families prefer to keep contacts to a minimum; they do not like being reminded of the illness. Eventually, as the patient deteriorates, weekly and then daily visits will usually be needed and welcomed.

Table 9.1   Strategies for promoting home care

1. Maintain regular contact.
2. Availability of support and advice 24 hours day, 7 days a week.
3. Elicit and address fears and concerns.
4. Develop and rehearse plans to manage existing or anticipated problems.
5. Encourage and reinforce the carers efforts.
6. Involve other agencies in easing the burden of care, when appropriate.
7. Consider an alternative place of care as a backup option.
8. Consider respite care if illness is protracted.
9. Teach families about the signs of the terminal phase.

Availability of Support and Advice Twenty-four Hours a Day, Seven Days a Week

There should be some way for patients and families to get urgent advice and support between visits. This is particularly important if problems arise during the night or at weekends. Very often, they will only want reassurance about a minor problem such as a subtle change in the patient's condition. This is especially likely to happen at night, when time seems to drag and people are most vulnerable. However, without reassurance, the problem will become magnified, taking on all of the anxieties and difficulties associated with home care.

Effective after-hours support can only be given if there is continuity of care from the health-care professionals. Some doctors choose to give their home telephone numbers to families; this privilege is rarely abused. When group practices are involved, it is important to make sure that partners are aware of the situation. Very ill patients have difficulty meeting new people. If continuity cannot be maintained, for example, if the family physician is going on holiday, then the person who is providing cover should be introduced as soon as possible Specialist palliative home-care teams often provide 24 hour cover. Whatever support is available, families should have clear written guidelines about who to contact, particularly after hours and at weekends.

Eliciting and Addressing Fears and Concerns

Time is needed to allow people to express their fears about being at home. Whenever the patient or carer appears anxious, check what is causing the anxiety. The temptation will be to reassure as soon as the problem is mentioned. However, the expressed concern often masks deeper worries which lie at the heart of whether it will be possible to cope. If people find it hard to be specific, then it can be helpful to ask 'What do you think is the worst thing that could happen?'. Because it takes time to get at these issues and to develop a response, visits must be planned to allow for this. This is where a multi-professional approach is helpful; nurse specialists often have more time for visits than physicians. However, careful co-ordination and liaison then becomes important in order to avoid duplication of service and over-burdening the patient and family.

When fears are ungrounded, correction of misinformation and reassurance may be all that is needed. Usually, the concerns are realistic. Even if the likelihood of the problem eventuating is remote, work on ways to overcome the problem rather than passing over it with reassurance. Whenever issues are discussed with the patient and family, check that they have understood what has been said, that the information has addressed their concerns, and that the information has not raised further questions or worries. If the subject has been a difficult one, for example, what will happen to the patient's waning appetite and energy, then a follow-up visit or telephone call is often worthwhile.

Young children and adolescents are often left out of these important conversations. Parents find it hard to respond to the needs of children; it is easier to assume that they are too young to understand. However, avoidance of the issues does not protect the patient or the main carer. Both continue to sense and observe the distress of the children struggling alone with their fears and fantasies. Children need support for their sadness. They need opportunities to express their feelings. They also need clear, simple information about what has happened and why, and what is likely to happen. Children often have specific worries about their own future. For example, they may need reassurance that the family will survive, that they have not caused the patient's illness, that they themselves will not become ill, or that the surviving parent is not going to die as well.

Parents usually need some preparation before the needs of children can be addressed. If the subject is not raised then a question such as 'How do you think the children are coping?' will often elicit the concerns, the examples of queries from the children which show they do have needs, the feelings of helplessness at not knowing how to respond, and the fear that dealing with these needs will make the children feel worse. Sometimes, the worry is that confronting the children's needs will make the patient worse, particularly if the patient is trying desperately to deny the illness. Having established what the issues are, it is then possible to affirm that the children do have needs and that meeting these needs will benefit rather than destroy their emotional integrity. While some of the issues raised will be painful, working through them will make things easier, not just for the children but also for the parents. Sometimes, reassurance and advice is sufficient to enable the parents to take control, otherwise a health-care professional will need to facilitate the process.

Developing and Rehearsing Plans to Manage Existing or Anticipated Problems

Too often, health-care professionals are used to taking control of problems on behalf of patients and families. At home, this only reinforces families' fears that they cannot provide adequate care. When something goes wrong and a health-care professional is not available, the patient will then end up being admitted to hospital. In a recent study comparing hospital and hospice admissions, more than half of the patients who died in hospital were admitted as emergencies, with either the general practitioner or the family calling for an urgent ambulance (Seale and Kelly, 1997).

Many families can be better trained to care. Empowering lay carers requires that health-care professionals deliberately hand over knowledge and skills, according to the needs and capabilities of the relatives. This process requires time and patience. Two common problems – pain and the fear of the patient falling – will serve to illustrate how this can be achieved. Pain is a common symptom. If the patient is not already experiencing pain then he is likely to; more significantly, the patient and the family will think he is likely to. Having clarified any misconceptions that the patient and family might have, for example, that pain will kill the patient, the next step is to devise a plan with them. The plan should consist of simple, logical steps which are clearly written down: if pain occurs or gets worse, take a specified amount of pain killer such as 10 ml of morphine elixir, check that the pain is relieved after a specified time, if not then repeat the dose of pain killer, until the pain is relieved. The plan should include a contact number if further advice or support is needed at the time. Appropriate contingencies should be considered, such as having suppositories available if nausea or vomiting is expected. If the patient is receiving medication via a syringe pump, the family should still have some means of dealing with break-through pain. This same process should be applied to any other actual or potential symptoms.

The written plan will not be sufficient. The implementation of the plan should be rehearsed with the patient and family, often on several occasions. This is especially important when they need to learn new skills, for example, how to give suppositories or how to use equipment. As with any new skill, hands-on practice is needed to supplement written or verbal instructions. Syringe pumps are often used for dying patients at home. Family carers can often be trained to change the syringes. This will increase their sense of involvement and reduce the feelings of helplessness. Not every relative will want to, and it should not be imposed.

Ideally, the process of training in pain control should start even before the patient is discharged home. Too often, medications are started in the hospital setting without consideration of how the patient and family will manage at home. For example, a patient with pancreatic carcinoma was sent home with pain controlled by slow-release morphine tablets. Within 24 hours, there was a telephone call from the distressed husband that his wife was in unbearable pain. When the home-care team arrived, it was clear that he had not given the extra morphine for break-through pain as instructed. He was too frightened to give the morphine elixir because his hands were so unsteady that he was not able to pour out 15 ml accurately. He was afraid that he would overdose his wife. When the husband was reassured that a few millitres extra was not a danger, he managed future episodes of break-through pain with confidence.

The fear of the patient having a fall is common. It is a realistic fear when the patient is weak and unsteady. Even if the carer does not raise the issue, it is often worth discussing. As with symptom control, a written plan is often helpful. The carer should be discouraged from attempting to lift the patient. It is easier to make the patient comfortable on the floor with a pillow and blanket if necessary. Then the carer should contact people who have been asked and are prepared to help get the patient back into bed. This might include neighbours, other family, or health-care professionals such as community nurses or ambulance crew. Carers often feel reluctant to ask neighbours or family but it is surprising how often they want to help, easing their own sense of helplessness.

Whenever possible, ways should be found to involve children in the care. This may just be preparing food or helping with other simple physical tasks. Older children can benefit from the responsibility and training about managing pain, etc. This can free the main carer to take short breaks, giving the child the satisfaction of helping both parents.

Encouraging and Reinforcing the Carers' Efforts

Even with carefully prepared plans, carers still need a lot of support and encouragement. The burden of responsibility can be eased if their efforts are praised appropriately. Whenever a contact or a visit is made, check whether the plan has needed actioning. Even if the carer's response was not quite according to plan, for example, a follow-up dose of analgesic is not given when the first dose is not effective, give praise for what was done. Then find out what made it difficult to follow through the plan: was the carer worried, is the plan realistic, etc? Using the carer's feedback to amend the plan will further enhance self-esteem and confidence. Spontaneous encouragement at other times is also helpful. When leaving the house, for example, a genuine comment such as 'I am very impressed with the care that you are providing' will help.

While positive feedback is helpful, it can discourage carers from saying how they really feel. Relatives should be given opportunities to vent negative feelings about caring, such as anger and guilt. They need reassurance that these feelings are normal and do not mean that they have stopped loving the patient.

Involving Other Agencies in Easing the Burden of Care, when Appropriate

The physical burden of caring for a terminally ill patient at home can be very taxing, especially if the course of the illness is protracted. Fatigue and exhaustion may actually cause the relative to become physically ill. There are many services that can help with the physical care, such as district nurses, home help agencies, meals-on-wheels, community occupational therapists and physiotherapists, and dieticians. The use of these services has to be discussed sensitively with the patient and carer lest the offer be interpreted as a sign of failure on the part of the carer. There is a difficult balance between introducing services early enough so that relationships can be formed but not so early that patient and family are offended. Another difficult problem is bringing in services to support the carer when the patient refuses to have them. This situation requires careful discussion and negotiation. The prospect of having to go into an institution if the carer becomes exhausted may be enough to swing the patient's decision. However, some patients stubbornly hold out, placing enormous emotional pressure on the carers. Then, frequent visits are needed to support the carer.

Considering Alternative Places of Care or Respite Care

Whenever the patient wants to die at home and the carer disagrees, it is helpful to identify an alternative place of care. Often the carer will broach the subject when the patient is not in the room: 'I do not want him to die at home. Please tell me when he is near the end so we can get him somewhere else'. In talking to the patient, acknowledge the patient's wishes ('I know that you want to be at home') but affirm what the carer is saying. Then, point out that the patient is more likely to stay at home longer if the carer knows that there is a fall-back option and invite the patient to choose. Anxious families will often cope better if there is a back-up plan, and it is even worth discussing it with families and patients who are determined for a home death 'just in case'. It is much easier to activate a hospice or hospital admission if things have been planned in advance.

Short periods of respite care, particularly when the illness is protracted, will help the family to rest and recuperate. Many hospice in-patient units offer short one- or two-week admissions for respite. Other services can provide respite at home, particularly at night. In the UK, the Marie Curie Nursing Service provides trained nurses for this purpose. Some palliative-care services in the community also have teams of trained nurses and assistants who can provide 'hands-on' care and support for longer periods during the day, supplementing the care from the district nurses.

Teaching Families about the Signs of the Terminal Phase

At some point before the patient starts to die, it is possible to teach families, and sometimes patients, about what happens during the terminal phase. Most carers will ask, although it may not be a direct question. They usually appreciate specific information. The common signs include:

1. Increasing lethargy, with the patient spending more time sleeping during the day. Avoid telling the family that death is like the patient falling asleep.
2. Decreasing appetite and then decreasing thirst. If carers are not prepared for these signs, there is often a crisis request for admission when the patient stops eating and drinking.
3. The patient will be unlikely to swallow tablets and other medicines. This means a syringe pump or suppositories might be needed.
4. Confusion may occur.
5. Incontinence.
6. Diminishing urine output if the patient is catheterised.
7. Noisy, 'rattling' breathing. The pattern of the breathing is often irregular, sometimes more rapid, often with long pauses.
8. Skin mottling and cooling of the peripheries.

During the final terminal phase, carers need to be aware of the pressure that can result from the increase in visitors and telephone calls. A helpful strategy is to nominate another relative who is contacted on a daily basis and who then updates everyone else on the patient's progress. This is also a time when family or friends suddenly turn up. Major problems can then ensue if old arguments or dysfunctional relationships are suddenly reactivated.

When the patient is dying, carers should be told about the signs of death: the patient will stop breathing, usually after a short period of 'sighing' or gasping respirations which occur at intervals up to one or two minutes, and cannot be roused by shaking or shouting. They will need reassuring that this process is usually peaceful, not loud or violent. It is better to warn them if this is not expected to be the case, for example, a patient who has premonitory bleeding from a fungating tumour eroding on to the carotid artery.

Specific instructions about what to do after the patient has died are also helpful. Carers may need to be told that they do not need to attempt resuscitation or dial for an ambulance. Emergency services are often compelled by policy to attempt resuscitation and take the patient to the nearest hospital. This will be extremely distressing to the family. The patient has to be pronounced dead by a medical practitioner. If the family physician is away, alternative arrangements should be made for death certification so that a coroner's inquest is avoided. There is no urgency about contacting an undertaker if the family want to spend time with the body. Carers may benefit from knowing what reactions to expect from others, for example, an extremely emotional outburst from a distraught relative, and how to facilitate the grief reactions of children.

Models of Community-Based Specialist Palliative-Care Services

Within two years of opening, St Christopher's Hospice developed the first specialist home-care service. The service was designed to work with the existing community-based services such as general practitioners and district nurses. Specialist nurses were trained to give advice and support but did not provide direct physical care. The home-care team also included doctors and social workers, with ready access to chaplaincy and physiotherapy from within the Hospice if needed. Patients and families can contact the service 24 hours a day, 7 days a week.

Since then, the number of home-care teams has grown rapidly in the UK, the United States and also in other countries. There are over 400 home-care teams in the UK. Many teams provide a similar pattern of advisory services to that set up by St Christopher's, though the interdisciplinary composition and the hours of working may vary. One third of the teams are linked to hospice in-patient services; many are stand-alone. In England, the Cancer Relief Macmillan Fund charity has provided money to 'pump-prime' community nurse specialist posts. Many appointments have been funded this way; the term 'Macmillan nurses' is now synonymous with community-based palliative-care nurse specialists.

In some countries, community-based palliative-care teams have to provide 'hands-on' care because generic nursing services are very limited. Another model is for generic community services to include palliative-care nurse specialists working alongside the district nurses. This has the disadvantage of leaving the nurse specialists relatively unsupported. Respite-care teams of nurses and volunteers are being increasingly used to provide more practical support for carers at home, sometimes referred to as 'hospice-at-home'.

Hospice In-Patient Units

Hospice in-patient units are dedicated to the care of terminally ill patients. Some hospices have free-standing buildings, either renovated or purpose built. Community fundraising is often used to provide these facilities. Other hospice units have developed within acute hospitals. They are also known as palliative-care units. All or part of a ward is often adapted to provide terminal care. Sometimes, a separate building will be established in the grounds of the hospital. Palliative-care units are more likely to be funded from non-charitable sources which fund the hospital. An important characteristic of hospice units is the common purpose of the staff. Team-working is the norm. Clinical and other meetings are designed to facilitate this. The multidisciplinary team comprising medical, nursing, chaplaincy and other paramedical staff are dedicated to providing palliative care. Volunteers play an important part, particularly in the hospices funded by charitable donations. The ratio of staff to patients is deliberately kept at higher levels to allow more time for care and support of the patients and families. Hospices place a lot of emphasis on training staff and volunteers.

Hospice and palliative-care units pay careful attention to the physical environment. Landscaping is often used to supplement the interior decor. The aim is to create a restful, therapeutic environment which is balanced with the need to maintain an efficient clinical service. The challenge of achieving this aim often appeals to the community supporters of hospices. As a result, most units have furnishings and equipment which has been donated.

The population of patients served by hospices is highly selected. Almost all patients will have cancer, even in units which have a policy of accepting patients with non-malignant conditions. This reflects the greater uncertainty of predicting prognosis in patients who do not have cancer. Patients who are still receiving active treatments such as chemotherapy are often not accepted by hospices. There is no evidence to suggest that patients admitted to a hospice are more likely to come from particular socio-economic or religious backgrounds. There is an under-representation of patients from black and other minority ethnic groups.

The major determinant of whether a patient is admitted is whether or not the patient is given the choice. Most people are never given the option. In districts which have more beds, a greater proportion of cancer patients will be given the choice. At least half of the patients who are offered the option of admission will turn it down. They are frightened that a hospice is a place of no hope. This fear can be overcome if the patient and family meet palliative-care staff working in the community or in the hospital who can allay the misconceptions. Patients who are transferred to hospices against their will are likely to 'give up' and die very quickly (Dunlop et al., 1989).

In the UK, the average in-patient unit has between 10 and 16 beds. The range is from two beds in small hospitals up to 62 beds at St Christopher's and St

Joseph's Hospices. Overall, about 14% of all cancer deaths occur in hospices. This proportion is higher in areas where there are more beds. For example, one third of cancer deaths in the St Christopher's catchment area occur in the Hospice. Some smaller units specify a maximum length of stay, usually around two weeks. This is to avoid the hospice being used as an alternative to long-term nursing homes. The fact that hospices do not charge for their care makes this a very real possibility. Two or three patients staying for many months could seriously limit the number of admissions to a 7- or 10-bed unit. Larger units have a longer length of stay and are more likely to admit very elderly patients.

The main reason for admission to hospices is terminal care. Either the patient has no carer or the family are not able or willing to look after the patient at home. Palliative-care units in hospitals can be put under considerable pressure to admit dying patients from acute wards, thereby preventing the beds from being 'blocked' to routine or emergency admissions. Patients must be well enough to be transferred, otherwise they may die in transit or will not benefit from being in an unfamiliar environment with new staff.

Hospices also provide symptom control in difficult cases, particularly when the patient and family cannot manage at home. A short admission for intensive treatment and monitoring can often facilitate the patient's going home again. The other reason for admission is respite care to give the relatives a break from the physical burden of caring. Up to one third of admissions to hospices result in patients being discharged again.

Given that many patients die in hospices, staff have to be aware of the potential impact on the other patients, particularly those who stay for longer periods. Hospices are not maudlin, depressing places. Quite the contrary, visitors always comment on the relaxed, peaceful atmosphere which is in sharp contrast to acute hospitals. Many patients find it reassuring to see the comfortable way in which people die, but staff are trained to respond to any concerns that may arise.

Occasionally, some patients with a prognosis of several months are admitted to hospices. Larger hospices may intentionally take patients with conditions such as motor neurone disease. These patients are often too young to be considered for nursing homes. Their physical, emotional and spiritual needs are also better met in hospices which have greater staff:patient ratios. Some cancer patients require longer-term care. Examples include patients with paraplegia from spinal cord compression and patients who are severely disabled by intracerebral tumours. Special attention must be paid to the psychological impact of staying in a hospice, not just on the patient but also on the staff.

Hospices are always concerned about admitting people who would be more appropriately treated in nursing homes. Hospice care is free to the patient and family, in contrast to the expense of nursing-home care. The patient and family do not have to undergo any means testing or other rigorous social services evaluation before admission to a hospice. It is not surprising therefore that the diagnosis of cancer in a frail elderly person can be greeted with relief by health-care professionals. They can refer the patient to a hospice rather than try to get the patient transferred to a nursing home, with all the inherent delays that cause the hospital bed to be blocked. The desire to make a cancer diagnosis may lead to inappropriate decision making. For example, an abnormal chest x-ray may be considered sufficient to establish the diagnosis of cancer. When there is doubt, hospice staff will often review such patients before admission. It is better to identify that someone is not appropriate beforehand than to admit the person to a hospice and then have to transfer them to a nursing home, having already experienced the level of care in a hospice.

Day Hospices

The first day hospice was established at St Luke's Hospice in Sheffield in 1975. There are currently 230 day hospices in the UK. They provide a variety of activities and services for terminally ill people who are living in the community. Two thirds of day hospices are attached to in-patient units, which enables them to serve in-patients as well. Most people attend on a once- or twice-weekly basis. Indirectly, day hospices also support the carers, providing them with the chance for a break to do other things.

Day hospices seek to create an environment in which people can develop new relationships, new interests and exploit new opportunities, all with the purpose of enhancing quality of life. Volunteers often play an important role in this process, not just by providing transport, but also by befriending patients and supporting the various activities. Many of the activities centre around a mid-day meal which is prepared and served by the volunteers.

The services provided by day hospices vary from unit to unit. These will include: activities which encourage socialising such as card games; entertainment; complementary therapies such as massage and aromatherapy; art and music therapy; outings; and handicrafts. Some day hospices provide rehabilitation, lymphoedema bandaging, blood transfusions and other 'medical' services. The day hospice may serve as a clinic for medical reviews as well.

Not all patients are comfortable with the idea of attending a day hospice. For some, there are negative connotations, rightly or wrongly, linked with day-care facilities for the elderly. Others find it hard to meet new people or to travel when feeling weak and tired. However, for those patients who do attend, day hospice often becomes a highlight of the week.

Palliative Care in Acute Hospitals

Over 90% of cancer patients are never admitted to a hospital at some point in their illness. Even when specialist palliative-care services such as hospices and home-care teams are available, many patients die in acute hospitals. A prospective study of 100 cancer patients dying in hospital (Dunlop et al., 1989) showed that one third of patients were receiving active treatments, such as radiotherapy and chemotherapy, or were being investigated at the first presentation of advanced disease. A similar proportion chose to die in hospital, preferring not to be at home or to be transferred to a hospice. A recent study carried out by St Christopher's Hospice has shown that even those patients who were admitted to hospital as 'emergencies' and who were too ill to be transferred, would not have wanted hospice care. These patients and their families had not wanted to acknowledge the cancer diagnosis.

There are many factors which make it difficult to provide good palliative care in acute hospitals. The emphasis on diagnosis and cure has created a culture in which the death of a patient is seen as a failure. Even when more staff become aware of the importance of palliative care, they lack the resources and the training needed to deliver it. In the St Christopher's Hospice study referred to above, families of patients who died in hospitals were just as likely to have cared for the patient during the final admission as relatives of patients who died in the Hospice. However, the reasons for helping with the care were very different. In the Hospice, relatives wanted to help as a way of demonstrating their affection for the patient. In the hospital, relatives felt compelled to help because they felt that the patients were not getting adequate care owing to staff shortages.

The care of dying patients is often relegated to the nurses and the junior medical staff. Both sets of professionals feel inadequately trained. In the case of doctors, few medical schools have more than one or two days for teaching on pain control and palliative care. Communication skills are being taught more often but the pressure on already crowded undergraduate curriculae is growing constantly. Doctors are rarely taught how to make the difficult decisions about stopping unnecessary treatments for people who are dying. The stress of these decisions adds to the sense of helplessness in the face of uncontrolled symptoms and the anguish of patients and relatives. In the absence of formal support systems, it is little wonder that doctors avoid the dying, fail to detect symptoms and over-report anxiety as a problem for relatives.

Nurses are involved with terminally ill patients from the beginning of their career on the wards. In nurse training, more teaching is now available on aspects of palliative care. However, whatever training they get in symptom control, for example, will be undermined if there is no support from the doctors. Nurses are more likely to be exposed to the distress of the relatives, especially when doctors disagree about, or are unclear about, treatment decisions. Nurses frequently lack support from other staff, including other nurses and supervisors, in coping with this distress.

Hospices have had an indirect effect on improving care in hospitals. Hospice staff often teach students. Nursing staff who have worked in hospices may go back to work in the acute setting. Palliative-care units provide even more opportunities for training and work experience, especially if they are based in the same buildings as the hospital. However, despite these indirect effects, there are still major problems in providing palliative care in hospitals. These problems have led to the development of another very important specialist palliative-care service: the hospital-based advisory palliative-care team.

Hospital-Based Advisory Palliative-Care Teams

The concept of a specialist advisory service within the hospital was established in the mid-1970s. They were initially known by a variety of names: support-care teams, support teams and symptom-control teams. Palliative-care team is now the most widely used. The first team in the UK was set up in St Thomas' Hospital. The value of these teams was only slowly recognised. In 1977, there were two such teams. By 1989, this number had only grown to 38. In the past five years there has been a rapid expansion, largely due to the 'pump-priming' money available from the Cancer Relief Macmillan Fund. This has enabled more NHS hospitals to start up teams and there are even nurse specialists advising in private hospitals as well. There are now over 200 teams listed in the Hospice Information Service directory.

Palliative-care teams are multidisciplinary teams, comprising nurse specialists, doctors and other staff such as social workers. The exact composition varies from hospital to hospital but the common theme is that the team does not have direct control of beds. The team members seek to improve palliative care by advising and supporting the ward staff. They do this in four ways:

1. Assisting in the relief of distressing symptoms and giving emotional, social and spiritual support to terminally ill patients.
2. Providing counselling and support for relatives.
3. Providing support and advice to staff caring for these patients and families.
4. Providing multidisciplinary education and training programmes.

Most teams do not operate a 24 hour on-call service. Close liaison is maintained with other specialist palliative-care services outside the hospital. Hospices and home-care teams can expedite the discharge of patients from hospital, as well as provide support and encouragement for the team members. Some hospital-based teams do operate within the community as well but this can detract from the work in the hospital.

Working in an advisory role can be very satisfying and very stressful. When hospital staff welcome the advice, the care of patients and families will improve noticeably. However, not all staff are so encouraging, especially when the team is newly established. Colleagues in other services that are suffering cost cut-backs may deeply resent the appearance of a new service. This underlines the importance of carefully planning and marketing a team before and after it starts. Other health-care professionals will feel affronted or threatened by the implicit criticism of existing services inherent in setting up a team. As a result, they will refuse to accept advice, leaving the patient, family and other staff even more distressed. This is doubly hard for team members who have trained in hospices and are used to being in control of the patients' care.

Vision and perseverance are needed to overcome the difficulties of the advisory role. If the issues are confronted head on, the care of the patient is likely to suffer. More importantly, the future care of other patients will be threatened as well; they will not be referred to the team. The team members must control their anger and frustration while making diplomatic attempts to improve the situation. Sometimes, a 'wait and see' approach is best; it is surprising how often advice is taken afterwards. At other times, dialogue and compromise are needed. Rarely is it necessary to abandon the situation completely. Whenever efforts are made by the medical or surgical team in favour of the patient, liberal praise should be given. Ultimately however, it is the degree of compromise that team members will accept that will determine whether they can survive the rigors of working in this way.

Palliative Care and Long-Term-Care Settings

With the increasing population of the very elderly, more people need care in nursing homes and other long-term-care institutions. Despite the advanced age of nursing home residents, only a relatively small proportion die of cancer. This reflects the falling incidence of cancer in the ninth and tenth decades. Those very elderly cancer patients with a short prognosis are more likely to die in hospital or in a hospice.

For long-term residents who do develop cancer, the standards of care are variable. Health-care professionals often believe that elderly patients do not experience pain or do not need such strong pain-killers. It can be very difficult to know if a demented or confused patient is experiencing pain. The low staff numbers and their lack of training mitigate against good palliative care. Up to one third of very elderly residents with cancer who experience pain will not be given analgesics; only a small minority get adequate pain-killers (Mor et al., in press). More training is needed for nursing staff and for the doctors who provide medical backup for nursing homes. Additional support and advice can be available from specialist home-care teams who help manage the patient as if he or she were at home.

Palliative Care and Specialist Cancer Treatment Services

Modern anti-cancer therapies are becoming increasingly sophisticated. New treatments are constantly being discovered and evaluated. Surgical techniques now include cryotherapy, laser therapy and reconstruction, for example. Radiotherapy machines can deliver a broader range of treatments with greater accuracy and fewer side-effects. More chemotherapeutic agents are available, along with biological response modifiers and hormone therapies. The evaluation of patients for these treatments requires the use of more accurate imaging and diagnostic techniques. Treatments are often given in combination, which requires careful planning and co-ordination. All of these factors have led to the development of specialist cancer-treatment centres where experts from the various oncology, radiotherapy, pathology and other related disciplines work together.

Despite the many advances, the majority of the major cancers remain incurable. It is still difficult to detect many cancers early enough to effect cure. The development of resistance to treatments such as chemotherapy often makes eradication of unresectable disease impossible. Oncologists are becoming more aware of quality of life issues when planning treatments for this group of patients. However, the recent ECOG study (Cleeland et al., 1994) illustrates how difficult it is for oncologists to deal with the symptoms of advancing cancer such as pain.

There is greater recognition by clinicians and health-care planners that cancer-treatment services and palliative-care services need to be linked together.

The early involvement of palliative-care services will give patients more options of symptom control and psycho-social support while they have anti-cancer therapy. This encourages lower morbidity during treatment. It also improves continuity of care, particularly when patients enter the terminal phase of the illness. There is less shock and dislocation when the anti-cancer treatments are no longer working. The emphasis of palliative care on the 'whole' patient and the family further enhances the care which is delivered. The easy flow of patients between the various treatment settings can be very efficient as well as empowering. Palliative-care services in the community can link with the hospital, with the primary health-care team and with the hospice, to the benefit of all concerned.

Palliative-care physicians can benefit by working alongside cancer specialists. They gain a better understanding of the biology of cancer and the treatments that are available. This can help identify patients who are referred directly to palliative-care services but should be considered for treatment. Cancer specialists have a rigorous approach to the diagnosis, staging and treatment of cancer, an approach which can improve the clinical skills of palliative-care physicians.

The biggest problem in collaborative working for palliative-care physicians is the nature of some treatments. The philosophical basis of palliative care has been to maximise quality of life, which also means minimising treatments that cause physical and psychological morbidity. It can be hard enough watching the effects of curative treatments such as bone marrow transplantation or multi-drug chemotherapy for high-grade lymphomas. However, more radical treatments are being attempted for 'incurable' cancers, such as high-dose chemotherapy and bone marrow transplantation for breast cancer. The abhorrence for these treatments will prevent palliative-care practitioners from realising that patients themselves will often go to extreme lengths, taking even the smallest chance of cure. By accepting the wishes of patients, and by supporting them with the skills and expertise of palliative medicine, the paradox is that many more patients and families can be helped to come to terms with their diagnosis.

Conclusion

This chapter has highlighted the various ways in which the principles of palliative care have been adapted to different care settings. In this age of cost-effectiveness in health care, the question is often asked: 'How effective are these services?'. This raises issues about cost and the quality of these services. These issues are examined in the next chapter.

10 – Evaluation of Palliative-Care Services

Introduction

Dame Cicely Saunders recognised the importance of evaluating palliative-care services when St Christopher's Hospice was founded. The financial considerations were a factor. Potential donors had to be convinced of the value of palliative care. However, it was even more important to establish the credibility of this entirely new field of medicine. If the principles of palliative care were to be established in general medical practice, they had to be backed up by sound, high-quality research. The rapid growth of palliative care and its spread throughout the world testifies to the wisdom of Dame Cicely's foresight.

Ongoing evaluation of palliative care is still needed. As a new specialty, palliative care emerged into a time when the funding of health care was changing throughout the western world. The escalating costs of technological advances in diagnostic and therapeutic treatments have caused pressure on government funding of health-care services. New palliative-care programmes have to compete for money alongside existing medical and surgical services. Established hospices have to demonstrate their effectiveness and efficiency to preserve contracts with funding authorities. As more information about cancer is made available to the public, the expectations of patients and families is increasing. Palliative care needs to adapt services to meet these expectations. The limitations of current symptom-control treatments need to be identified so that improvements can be made. New treatments which are developed need to be tested against existing options.

The assessment of a service depends on measuring outcomes of care. An outcome is defined as any change in patients' health status which can be attributed to treatment or care. Information about outcomes is keenly desired by health-care planners so that different treatments and different health-care delivery systems can be compared. When this information is combined with cost comparisons, rational decisions can be made about the allocation of health-care resources. This possibility has encouraged a burgeoning number of studies and meta-analyses for evaluating care, as well as methodologies to use this knowledge for rationing purposes.

Palliative care has the broad aim of maximising quality of life for patients with progressive cancer and their families. Several outcomes of care relate to the concept of quality of life; this chapter begins by reviewing how the concept is defined. The problems in measuring these outcomes are outlined. The studies which have compared palliative-care services with conventional care are described. The cost implications are then considered. The chapter concludes by considering the role of clinical audit in evaluating palliative-care services.

What is Quality of Life?

In business and manufacturing, a quality product is often thought of as expensive, reliable, beautiful and luxurious. It has been assumed that these characteristics represent an absolute standard, below which a product could not be considered as being a quality product. However, customers have widely differing views about what is beautiful, what is desirable. Therefore, quality-assurance experts recommend that a quality product should be judged on whether it conforms to the customers' expectations (Crosby, 1976). For example, an expensive car would be expected to have all the characteristics described above, but a cheaper vehicle might still be a quality product because it is more accessible and because peoples' expectations of what the product offers are lower.

The customer perspective on quality has been carried over into health-care research. Several investigators, such as Spitzer et al. (1981), Padilla et al. (1990) and MacAdam and Smith (1987), have used focus groups to find out what constitutes quality of life for patients with advanced cancer. Most groups have included relatives of patients, along with other members of the public drawn from a variety of backgrounds. All of these studies have confirmed that quality of life is not a simple entity but a complex multifactorial concept. Some common themes have emerged.

Spitzer et al. (1981) used three panels of 43 people, including four cancer patients and four relatives in each panel. The panels proposed several characteristics of quality of life, which were refined after discussion with 217 cancer patients, and then presented to another panel of lay people including patients with cancer. Five items were chosen as measures of quality of life: involvement in an occupation, activities of daily living, perceptions of personal health, support of family and friends, and outlook on life.

Padilla et al. (1990) interviewed cancer patients who were experiencing pain. The patients were asked to define quality of life, what contributed to a good quality of life and to a bad quality of life, and how pain influenced their quality of life. Forty-one subjects were interviewed, by which point minimal new information was being obtained. Not surprisingly, pain was the most important factor which interfered with quality of life, both the physical pain and, more importantly, the meaning of the pain. Other symptoms also had negative effects, especially feeling weak and being unable to concentrate. Psychological experiences could also detract from quality of life, for example, feelings of insecurity, inner turmoil and not being successful in life. The capacity to enjoy a normal life, to remain independent and to work, were all highly rated. Social relationships were also important. Quality of life was diminished if family were unsupportive, if patients felt they were making others unhappy or not fulfilling their usual roles.

MacAdam and Smith (1987) used the same methodology as Spitzer et al.

(1981) to develop a questionnaire. Their phase one group comprised 30 people including one patient with terminal cancer and two relatives of deceased patients. The draft questionnaire was presented to 259 cancer patients who were also asked open-ended questions about their main concerns. The domains of quality of life which were then incorporated in the questionnaire were symptoms, mood, worries about family, fears about the future, knowledge about the illness and the degree of support.

Family members are also affected by quality of life issues but much less work has been done in this area. Kristjansen (1986) has interviewed many relatives of terminally ill cancer patients. She found that caring had physical and psychological consequences which affected their quality of life. Social and financial problems also had adverse effects. As with patients, the impact of any specific quality of life issue varied for each individual family member.

Table 10.1 summarises the variety of domains that contribute to quality of life.

Table 10.1   Dimensions of quality of life (after Bergner et al., 1981)

1. Symptoms
2. Functional status
   (a) Self care
   (b) Mobility
   (c) Physical activity
3. Role activities
   (a) Work
   (b) Household management
4. Social functioning
   (a) Personal interactions
   (b) Intimacy
   (c) Community interactions
5. Emotional status
   (a) Anxiety
   (b) Stress
   (c) Depression
   (d) Locus of control
   (e) Spritual well-being
6. Cognition
7. Sleep and rest
8. Energy and vitality
9. Health perceptions
10. General life satisfactions

The multi-dimensional nature of quality of life means that outcome studies must specify which domains are relevant. For research purposes, quality of life has to be defined by the investigators in the context of the study. Studies about the impact of hospice care have so far addressed the following quality of life dimensions: pain control, control of other symptoms and performance status; satisfaction with care; patients' psycho-social outcomes; and the physical and psycho-social experiences of family members before and after the death of the patient. The other important outcome that has been studied is place of death, which has an effect on relatives' quality of life. It is often quoted that a home death is highly desirable, especially for patients. Some studies have attempted to link outcomes to cost.

Measuring Quality of Life in Cancer Patients

The design and construction of valid, reliable instruments which measure quality of life is a lengthy and demanding process. The ideal is to develop a 'gold standard' tool that is simple to use but can assess the variety of domains that are involved. In practice, several tools have been produced, each of which has a different emphasis. Table 10.2 lists some of the instruments which have been used to assess quality of life in cancer patients.

Table 10.2   Quality of life instruments for use with cancer patients

Scale	Domains covered				
	Functional status	Pain	Other symptoms	Psycho-social	Global
Karnofsky Index	×				
ECOG Performance Scale	×				
SEIQOL	×	×	×	×	
EORTC QLQ-30 Questionnaire	×	×	×	×	×
McGill Pain Questionnaire		×			
Memorial Pain Assessment Card (MPAC)		×			
Brief Pain Inventory		×			
Symptom Distress Scale		×	×		
Rotterdam Symptom Checklist		×	×	×	
Functional Living Index for Cancer (FLI-C)		×	×	×	
City of Hope Medical Center QL Survey		×	×	×	
'Macadam' Short 20-Part Questionnaire		×	×	×	
MOS Short-Form General Health Survey		×	×	×	
Hospital Anxiety and Depression (HAD) Scale				×	
Profile of Mood States (POMS) – short version				×	
Spitzer Quality-of-Life Scales				×	×

These instruments can be considered under the following headings.

Functional Status

The two most commonly used tools which have been used to assess patients' functional status are the Karnofsky Index (Schag et al., 1984) and the ECOG Performance Scale (Zubrod et al., 1960). They have the advantages of being short (the former has an 11 point scale and the latter uses a five-grade scale) and easily administered by staff. Physical function correlates with many other dimensions of quality of life. As one might expect, patients who are too weak to be independent are likely to feel more depressed, for example.

Symptom Distress

Pain assessment has been a major focus for research. This reflects how frequently it occurs in cancer patients, how much it is feared and the fact that there are many treatments available. The McGill Pain Questionnaire is regarded as the 'gold standard' for assessing pain. It measures pain site and intensity, as well as qualitative descriptors. The original version is too lengthy for use with terminally ill patients and a shortened version has been developed (Deschamps et al., 1992). The Memorial Pain Assessment Card (MPAC) has been validated for hospitalised cancer patients (Fishman et al., 1987). The card combines visual analogue scales and descriptors, and is very easy to use. The degree of pain relief is an important measure that was introduced with MPAC. Brief Pain Inventory is a longer instrument which analyses pain intensity, pain relief and the effects of pain in more detail.

Several scales have been developed to assess other symptoms and symptom distress. Many of these instruments also cover psycho-social issues and are therefore considered below in the section on multidimensional assessments. However, one of the earliest examples was the Symptom Distress Scale (McCorkle and Young, 1978). The 13 items included breathlessness, nausea, vomiting and bowel function, as well as pain.

Other investigators have used visual analogue scales (VASs) or Likert scales to measure specific symptoms. VASs comprise a horizontal or vertical line which is 100 mm long. At both ends there are statements about the symptom, for example, 'No pain' at one end and 'Worst imaginable pain' at the other end. The patient makes a mark on the line to indicate his perception of the pain intensity. The distance of the mark from the 'No pain' end is used for analysing responses. Other symptoms can easily be substituted for pain, such as 'No nausea' versus 'Worst imaginable nausea'. VASs are easy to administer but some patients have major problems understanding how to use them. Likert scales use descriptors such as 'mild', 'moderate', 'severe', 'intolerable' to grade the intensity of a symptom. This approach is often easier for patients to comprehend.

Psycho-Social Measures

Two instruments have been used specifically to assess psycho-social issues. The Hospital Anxiety and Depression Scale (HAD) (Zigmond and Smith, 1983) was originally developed for non-cancer populations. HAD was designed to exclude physical symptoms from the assessment of depression in particular. This makes it more useful for cancer patients because the emotional components of depression and anxiety are separated from the somatic manifestations which resemble the effects of cancer. It is easy to administer and score; there is ongoing work to establish the threshold scores for identifying anxiety and depression in terminally ill patients. The other instrument is a shortened 14-item version of the Profile of Mood States (POMS), designed to assess mood states and changes in mood. The shortened version has been developed specifically for patients with advanced cancer (Guadagnoli and Mor, 1989).

Multidimensional Assessments

There have been many questionnaires which comprehensively cover both physical and psycho-social issues. However, many of these are too time consuming for ill patients to complete. Some of the tools which are practical were produced to compare the toxicity and morbidity of chemotherapy regimens. The Rotterdam Symptom Check List assesses 30 symptoms and has eight scales to assess daily activities. It is well validated with a high sensitivity and specificity, is easily administered and rapidly scored (De Haes et al., 1990). Because it has been designed for the oncology setting, some items not appropriate in palliative-care settings and only some pain problems are covered: sore muscles, low back pain, headaches, abdominal ache and sore mouth. The Functional Living Index for Cancer (FLI-C) uses a linear analogue format and covers physical symptoms and activity, mood, work and social interaction (Schipper et al., 1984). The City of Hope Medical Center QL Survey also uses VASs for the 28 multi-dimensional items (Grant et al., 1990). Both instruments are easy to use, administer and score, but they are more appropriate for the oncology setting.

A questionnaire designed specifically to assess suffering in terminal illness was developed by MacAdam and Smith (1987). As described above, a systematic methodology was used to define the content. After early trials, a shortened version containing 20 items, including physical symptoms and psycho-social domains, was found to be suitable for routine use during the initial assessment by a professional. It emphasises the patients' perception of their needs and avoids multiple assessments by different disciplines within the palliative-care team.

The Spitzer QL Index (Spitzer et al., 1981) was carefully developed using feedback from cancer patients and their relatives. Five items assess physical activity, daily living, perception of own health, support from family and friends, and outlook on life. It is designed for use by physicians to assess specifically the relative benefits and risks of various treatments for serious illness. The validity of this instrument for terminally ill patients has been questioned.

The EORTC QLQ core questionnaire has been designed to measure multiple dimensions of quality of life in a heterogeneous group of cancer patients (Aaronson et al., 1993). The dimensions include physical functioning, symptoms of disease, side-effects of treatment, psychological distress, social interaction and global quality of life. The two-page questionnaire takes about 10 minutes to administer and has been shown to be valid and reliable. The group responsible for the core questionnaire are also developing modular questionnaires for specific cancer types, such as lung cancer, or outcomes such as sexuality, body image and satisfaction with medical care. The core questionnaire has been used in palliative care but a specific module is currently under development.

The Medical Outcomes Study Short-Form 36 (MOS–SF36) is an example of a generic multidimensional questionnaire that was designed to be used in all clinical settings, not just with cancer patients (Steward et al., 1988). It has been used to study cancer treatments but has limited applicability to specialist palliative-care services.

Global Quality of Life Scales

Spitzer et al. (1981) also developed a global measure of quality of life. It is a VAS which is very easy to complete. While a global score seems to simplify the problems of having to measure multiple dimensions, it does not replace the need to do so. It is not just a summation of these dimensions but probably represents a separate concept. The EORTC core questionnaire includes the global measure alongside the other items.

Difficulties in Evaluating the Effect Palliative-Care Services on Quality of Life

Aside from the difficulty of defining quality of life, there are several research issues which have complicated the evaluation of quality of life in palliative care. There are several issues regarding the validity and reliability of quality of life measures. When research was first carried out on terminally ill patients, instruments were used which had been developed for other patient populations. Several difficulties were encountered, for example, the physical symptoms of advanced cancer rendered invalid tools designed to measure mood and depression. Furthermore, there were more serious problems with response burden causing selection bias. Questionnaires which are long and comprehensive cannot be completed by very ill patients. Mor (1986) described the magnitude of these problems in the National Hospice Study of 1457 patients. In the last month of life, when patients are most symptomatic (experiencing up to 5.5 symptoms on average), there is a significant decrease in the response rate to questionnaires. Only two thirds of patients could respond at three weeks prior to death, decreasing to only one third at the last interview. The main reason for these problems was increasing cognitive impairment – only one third of patients had full mental faculties at the last interview. By using proxy respondents on behalf of the patients, Mor found that the non-responders were more likely to be symptomatic. Therefore, the group of patients for whom interventions are most important are the least accessible for the purposes of evaluating the treatments.

Several methods have been used to get around these problems. One approach was to develop shorter instruments, such as the five-item Spitzer Quality of Life scale, or to develop shorter versions of existing instruments, such as POMSs and the McGill Pain Questionnaire. Another approach was to use proxy respondents for patients, either a family member or professional staff caring for the patient. However, the assessments made by relatives bear only moderate correlation with patient assessments at best. They tend to overate the severity and distress of patients' symptoms and underestimate patients' satisfaction with life. Using staff members as proxies is complicated by their vested interest in minimising the unresolved problems experienced by the patient, especially if these problems are seen as a reflection on their care.

In palliative-care settings, the average length of stay is relatively short, often a matter of days to weeks. This compounds the problem of obtaining meaningful quality-of-life data from these very ill patients. Mor (1986) suggested a model for deciding which aspects of hospice patients' quality of life should be measured. Performance status and cognitive functioning are most profoundly affected and characterise the patients' decline. These aspects can be assessed by a family or staff member in contact with the patient for long periods. Pain and symptom control are the next important element which can be relatively easily assessed. Only when good symptom control has been achieved can meaningful improvement in psycho-social aspects be attempted.

Some fundamental criticisms have been raised about the existing quality-of-life instruments with respect to palliative care. Most quality-of-life measurements get worse in cancer patients as the disease progresses. Indeed, one of the measures of validity used in testing the EORTC core questionnaire was that scores would deteriorate when patients did not respond to anti-cancer treatments. Mount and Scott (1983) pointed out that some of these patients can experience significant improvements in quality of life which are not detectable with current measures. They quoted the example of a young man who described such experiences at a time when his scores on the Spitzer QL Index were appalling. This has led some investigators to begin developing instruments for existential and other issues that may be positively affected by palliative-care interventions.

Quality-of-life measurements are affected by the place in which the patient is receiving care. Patients in institutional settings are more likely to be compliant and responsive to interview questions because of their desire to please. A patient living at home is more likely to consider a visitor as an intrusion. In-patient units may be able to enrol more patients in studies but the findings are not necessarily transferable to the hospital or home setting. If records are used to obtain data, the ready availability of notes in in-patient settings compared with home care is another possible cause of bias.

A thorough evaluation of health-care outcomes requires comparison between different methods of health-care delivery. In palliative care, this is complicated by the difficulty of knowing at what point in the illness trajectory the patient's condition is being assessed. A patient who is near to death is likely to have more symptoms, to need more medication, and to experience more side-effects than a patient with a longer prognosis. The point at which a patient will die cannot be known prospectively, which means that measurements across different populations cannot be made at the same time in the course of the illness. This led Kane et al. (1981) to use a long prospective data-collection period. Other investigators have chosen to collect data prospectively and then analyse it after the patients have died. The date of death is used as time zero and the data is then examined at time intervals back from that point.

Another methodology is to compile retrospective data using the memories of carers after the patient has died. This approach has the advantage of random sampling of whole populations on the basis of death certification rather than place of care or place of death. The difficulties of selection bias can be overcome by this means. After a suitable period of bereavement, carers can recall details about service utilisation with some accuracy. However, their assessments of patients' symptoms are less reliable. It has already been noted that relatives over-estimate the severity of patients' pain when patients are still alive: relatives' responses follow a bell-shaped distribution which is skewed to the right of patients' distribution of responses. A different bias is encountered after bereavement. The distribution of relatives' assessments becomes polarised, the opposite of a normal distribution. Relatives tend to recall that patients either had minimal/no pain or had severe pain. Conclusions from such studies, particularly about symptom control, must be interpreted with caution.

The ideal method for studying whether different services produce a difference in the quality of life of patients is to conduct a multi-site randomised clinical trial using a treatment and a control group. There have been a small number of such studies but they have been very limited in their scope and general applicability. Each study has only taken place at one site and has tested different types of interventions with somewhat different results. Because the interventions tested were not similar, meta-analysis techniques across sites has not been possible. Recruitment to these studies was difficult; only a limited number of patients can be identified prospectively for accrual. Most investigators have concluded that the problems inherent in this type of study are too great ever to allow a large enough trial. Non-randomised studies have been more common but the methodological problems are greater. These studies can highlight important differences between groups but the transferability of these differences across all clinical settings is very limited.

Palliative-Care Outcomes

The most systematic and thorough review of palliative-care outcomes was undertaken by Mor and Masterton-Allen (1987). They conducted computer-assisted searches of medical, sociological, health planning, psychological and government documents sources. Over 2000 references were compiled and categorised to allow analysis of hospice outcomes. Despite the fact that the variety of studies, each with their own failings, had been carried out in different settings using different measures, Mor and Masterton-Allen felt that common themes could be identified. These themes are included in the following sections which examine components that make up palliative care. Additional conclusions of significant studies which have been published since 1987 have been included.

Pain Control

The modern hospice movement began by establishing the use of morphine for analgesia. Since then, there have been several studies on pain control. Parkes first compared the prevalence of severe pain in patients treated at St Christopher's Hospice with patients treated in nearby hospitals. He used the retrospective reports of surviving spouses and found that hospice patients were less likely to be in pain, were more likely to be mobile, but were not made more drowsy by the greater use of morphine. A follow-up study carried out 10 years later (Parkes and Parkes, 1984) found that levels of pain control were similar in hospice and hospital patients, suggesting that knowledge about pain control had disseminated from the hospice to the hospitals between the studies.

Two larger prospective studies have been less positive in their findings. Kane et al. (1984) conducted a randomised trial in which Veterans' Administration patients were assigned to receive care in a hospice or a hospital setting. He found no significant differences between experimental and control groups with regard to patients' ratings of pain intensity. The National Hospice Study was a non-randomised study conducted across several sites. Hundreds of patients were recruited from hospice home care, hospice in-patient units and high-quality hospital conventional care settings. The latter were selected oncology services. There were no differences in patients' ratings of pain between the various settings (Greer et al., 1988). When patients were too ill to self-report, family members reported that hospice patients were less likely to be in severe pain in the last month of life than non-hospice patients, although no more likely to be pain free.

The National Hospice Study results were criticised as not typifying the experience of patients cared for in less-expert non-hospice settings. The investigators were aware that the study had the effect of improving the level of pain assessment and control in the hospitals (Greer, personal communication). There have been two large studies published in the United Kingdom which have used large samples based on random analysis of death certificates from several health districts (Seale and Cartwright, 1994; Addington-Hall and McCarthy, 1995). Based upon the retrospective memories of relatives, there are significant differences in the proportion of patients who experience relief of pain in hospices versus acute hospitals.

There is some evidence that hospices may achieve significant improvements in pain control which can be translated into other settings. The differences are most pronounced when relatives report patients' condition because the patients' are too ill or have died.

Other Physical Symptoms

Terminally ill patients experience many symptoms other than pain. Although most effort has been directed at improving pain control, there are a wide range of strategies for treating symptoms such as breathlessness, nausea, vomiting and constipation. The problem in comparing the outcomes of different services is the relatively low prevalence of individual symptoms compared with the common occurrence of pain. Some studies have aggregated data for all symptoms but this still produced mixed results: some studies reporting no difference, other studies finding hospice benefits. The randomised study conducted by Kane et al. (1984) found no significant difference between the treatment and control groups in the number and severity of symptoms reported. The National Hospice Study found that families of patients reported a significantly lower number of different symptoms in the hospice group, but Mor and Masterton-Allan (1987) concluded 'that there was insufficient evidence to say that hospice care was more effective than conventional care in controlling patients' physical symptoms'.

Physical Functioning and Overall Quality of Life

Progressive cancer has a major effect on physical functioning. Patients become progressively weaker and more dependent. Although quality of life has psycho-social domains, these are affected by the ability to get about and interact socially. When a patient becomes weak, functional status and psycho-social attributes tend to decline in parallel. In the National Hospice Study, there were no differences in physical functioning and overall quality of life between the study groups. During the last month of life, most cancer patients became bedbound and dependent; these effects are very difficult to change.

Satisfaction with Care

Measuring satisfaction with health care is always difficult because few patients or relatives express dissatisfaction. Most surveys have found that patients and families in specialist palliative-care settings are more satisfied with the care than in hospitals. These findings have been replicated in the randomised studies that have been conducted. The Regional Study in the Care of the Dying also confirmed higher levels of relatives' satisfaction with specialist home care compared with district nursing services. Furthermore, Seale (1991) showed that when specialist home-care nurses worked with district nurses, the satisfaction of relatives with the care of district nurses was higher than when specialist nurses were not involved. Hospice services appear to deliver the kind of care which patients and families want, bearing in mind that not all patients and families choose these services.

Patient Psycho-Social Outcomes

Palliative care should improve patients' mood and sense of emotional well-being. This outcome is based on the principle of care for the whole person, rather than just treating the disease or the physical symptoms. The home-like ambience of hospice in-patient units should be more relaxing. Counselling and spiritual care should reduce depression, hopelessness and anxiety. Studies of psychological morbidities, such as anxiety and depression in terminally ill patients, indicate higher than normal levels of mood disturbance compared with normal controls. However, the levels of mood disturbance are still considerably less than for psychiatrically depressed patients. Hinton (1979) found that hospice patients were less depressed and anxious than hospital patients, who were more irritable. Other small non-randomised studies have also found less anxiety and worries in hospice patients.

In a study of specific psycho-social interventions for terminally ill patients, Linn et al. (1982) randomised patients to experimental and control groups. Patients in the experimental group were seen weekly, then monthly, for one year. The families were also seen. After three months, the patients who were counselled were less depressed, had higher self-esteem and higher life satisfaction than controls.

The Veterans' Administration Study did not find any differences in either depression or anxiety between hospice and control groups. The National Hospice Study also failed to demonstrate a difference in the study groups. When interpreting these results, Mor and Masterton-Allen (1987) drew attention to the variability of psycho-social interventions provided at the multiple sites in the study. They concluded that the hospice 'aura' and philosophy do not have an indirect effect on patients' emotional state. For positive effects, explicit interventions related to the hospice philosophy must be implemented.

Family Psycho-Social Outcomes

Most studies evaluating palliative care have looked at the effects on patients. Few have specifically reviewed the effect on family care-givers while the patient is still alive. In the Veterans' Administration Study, relatives of patients randomised to receive hospice care were less anxious than controls. There was no difference in the levels of depression. The National Hospice Study was able to look at the effects of home care. Not surprisingly, care-givers for patients at home contributed more to the direct care of patients. Despite this burden of care, there was no increase in levels of anxiety, depression or indirect evidence of psychological distress. These findings contrasted with the results of Parkes and Parkes' work (Parkes and Parkes, 1984). They found an increased level of psychological distress in relatives caring for patients at home. Seale and Kelly have recently completed a study (Seale and Kelly, 1997) comparing the experiences of relatives of patients who died in St Christopher's Hospice with nearby hospitals. He used the same methodology as Parkes used in previous studies. Both groups of relatives reported participating in the care of the patients in the hospice or in the hospital. However, the motivations for providing the care were different. In the hospice, relatives helped because they wanted to; in hospitals, some relatives felt they needed to help because of inadequate levels of staff and care.

Bereavement Care

Bereavement is often associated with physical and psychological morbidity in surviving relatives, especially spouses. The National Hospice Study followed all care-givers after the death of the patients. Carers of patients who died at home were more likely to report depression and anxiety. However, there were no significant differences for indirect measures of morbidity: rate of hospitalisation, number of visits to family physicians, use of alcohol or tranquillisers, and suicidal ideation. Other studies, reviewed by Parkes (1980), have compared the effects of bereavement counselling on selected bereaved with high-risk factors. In these studies, positive outcomes are evident. Bereavement services need to be focused to be effective.

Place of Death

Most cancer patients die in hospital, and the proportion of patients dying at home has declined progressively in recent decades. Overall, fewer than 30% of cancer patients now die at home. Mor and Masterton-Allen (1987) found that hospice programmes which emphasise home care will have 30%–70% of patients dying at home. They felt that this increase could not be explained solely on the basis of differences in patient characteristics and concluded that palliative-care services can facilitate home deaths for those patients and families who want it, whereas non-hospice services do not. Hospice in-patient units can also shift the place of death; opening a hospice in-patient unit will increase the proportion of hospice deaths while decreasing the proportion dying in hospital (Hill and Oliver, 1989). Hospital-based advisory palliative-care teams can also change the place of care. These teams increase the number of cancer patients discharged from hospital, particularly if there are strong links with community-based in-patient and home-care services.

Costs of Palliative-Care Services

As indicated above, surveys comparing palliative care with conventional care have shown that palliative care is certainly no worse, and in several respects confers benefits, on patients and families. Emanuel (1996) has provided the most recent review of the cost savings conferred by palliative-care services. He noted that the randomised Veterans' Administration trial showed no evidence of savings. However, non-randomised trials showed a wide range of savings, with increased savings in the last 6 months (10%–17%) and particularly the last month (25%–40%) of care. Savings were higher for home care compared with hospice in-patient services. In the United Kingdom, specialist palliative-care services are heavily subsidised from charitable sources such as donations and legacies. Approximately 60% of funding for hospice in-patient services is estimated to come from non-government sources. This further reduces the 'price' of care to the government compared with the cost of care.

With the greater potential for home care, cost savings from decreased hospital use may impose increased indirect costs on family care-givers. Using data from the National Hospice Study, Muurinen (1986) attempted to quantify this. He found that about half of carers had been in the labour force before the patients became ill – 27% of carers left work to care for the patient. This results in con-siderable lost earnings for these carers.

Auditing Palliative-Care Services

The systematic evaluation of palliative-care services has confirmed their place in the overall provision of health care. In the United States, the National Hospice Study contributed to the decision to provide government funding for hospice services through the Medicare hospice benefit. This funding has been available since the mid-1980s. In the United Kingdom, government planning and funding of palliative-care services has become increasingly explicit. The recent national review of cancer services emphasised the importance of collaboration between active cancer treatment centres and specialist palliative care. Contracts are now used as the basis for funding relationships between the health authorities and hospice services. Government agencies constantly need to justify expenditure, to ensure value for money. This means that health-care services must audit their activity; palliative care is no exception.

There are other important reasons for carrying out clinical audit, aside from ensuring the most effective use of resources. Patients and families are becoming more knowledgeable about health care. The Patient Charter is encouraging patients to demand higher standards of service. Some hospice services intrinsically feel that their service must be high quality simply because they are offering hospice care. This attitude can be deceiving and does not guarantee that outcome. Audit helps staff to be more focused, identifying and correcting problems in routine care which would otherwise be overlooked. Apart from the clinical benefits, audit can also highlight training and educational needs. For some disciplines, participation in clinical audit is a training requirement.

What is the Audit Process?

Audit is the systematic critical analysis of the quality of care. It is a cyclical process and, as such, should be ongoing. It begins with the observation of some aspect of clinical or organisational practice: structure, process or outcome. Structure refers to resource issues such as manpower numbers or composition, equipment, buildings or money. Process is the way in which the resources are organised and arranged to deliver care, for example, how often a home-care team meets together to discuss patient care and what procedures staff follow when admitting a patient. Outcome refers to the results of care and is the most important objective of the audit process. However, outcomes may be difficult to define and measure. This has led to a focus on process, with the assumption that if the process is right then the outcome will be right. It has also led to the mistake of confusing output with outcome. Output refers to the activity of an organisation, such as the number of people admitted to a hospice, the number of visits made by home-care nurses, etc. As with process, outputs do not necessarily correlate with outcomes. Whatever aspect of care is scrutinised, the measurements should be simple and straightforward, cause minimum disruption to the delivery of care, and should be made with valid and reliable instruments.

After the first stage of observation and description, the next phase of the audit cycle is to compare the care against some standard. Standards of care can be derived from the literature, obtained from professional organisations, or may be predetermined by the funding or monitoring agency. In the absence of a previous standard, the initial observations of care may serve to become a standard. Some standards have been developed as a consensus by professional representatives. The Trent Hospice Audit Group used senior medical and nursing representatives from hospices in the Trent region to create a set of core standards which are now being used to audit care.

When care is compared with a standard, deficiencies may be highlighted which need correction. If this happens, the final stage in the audit cycle is to implement changes to improve care. This has to be handled with skill and tact if staff are not to be left feeling threatened and hurt. The cycle is then repeated to ensure that the changes have worked. When care meets the standard, positive feedback and encouragement can be given to the staff. The aim is to make the audit cycle as interesting as possible, so that staff will never be satisfied with the current level of care and will be motivated constantly to seek improvements in care.

Introducing Clinical Audit

Higginson (1993) has given a clear, practical account of what is needed to introduce clinical audit. It is important to start with a commitment from management to the audit process. There is nothing more disheartening than identifying deficiencies in care only to find that appropriate resources and training will not be available for improvements. A group of clinical staff and managers should then meet and decide on a plan for audit. Palliative care requires a multidisciplinary approach, audit activities should involve the various disciplines. The audit cycle should start with small projects, followed up by regular meetings and feedback. Staff will be more committed if they can be involved in the process of setting and modifying standards, and if they see positive action taken to instigate changes.

The assessment process will depend on the clinical situation being reviewed. If it is patient or family care then some effort should be made to collect information from patients and families. Non-clinical staff who are not involved in patient care or decision making are often better placed to receive comments from patients, particularly if the comments might be critical. Volunteers with backgrounds as health-care professionals or in public relations can be used for this purpose, with appropriate training. Occasionally, it is helpful to get an external, independent view of the organisation, but this is usually very expensive.

Tools for Use in Clinical Audit

There is an increasing array of instruments which have been validated for and used in clinical audit of palliative care (see Table 10.3). Services which have used these instruments routinely find that patients' and families' problems are considered in more detail, there is a more systematic approach to the objectives of care and new staff readily learn what is required of them clinically.

Table 10.3   Tools for use in clinical audit

1. Support Team Assessment Schedule (STAS)
2. Edmonton Symptom Assessment Schedule (ESAS)
3. Palliative Care Core Standards
4. Retrospective views of bereaved relatives
5. Palliative Care Assessment (PACA) tool
6. Patient Evaluated Problem Score (PEPS)

Support Team Assessment Schedule (STAS)
STAS is an instrument designed to be rated by health-care professionals. There are several goals of care that are measured. The goals were developed after a literature review, patient and family interviews, and in collaboration with palliative-care services. Items cover physical, emotional and spiritual issues for patients and families, communication issues, and team effectiveness. It is widely used, having been adapted for use in several countries. STAS was originally designed for advisory community-based teams, but has been useful for hospice in-patient units and hospital-based teams as well. STAS has also been modified and used by non-specialist services, such as general practitioners and district nurses.

Edmonton Symptom Assessment Schedule (ESAS)
ESAS was originally developed in the palliative-care unit in Edmonton, Canada. It comprises nine VASs for measuring symptoms and psychological issues. There is also one blank VAS which can be defined by the patient. Scores are completed twice daily and reported in a graphical format. This allows trends and changes to be detected quickly. The patient usually fills out the VAS assessments but staff may help if the patient is unable to do it.

Palliative-Care Core Standards
As mentioned above, the Trent Hospice Audit Group have defined a set of core standards covering symptom control, emotional support, patient and carer information, bereavement care, collaboration between agencies and education for staff. The standards deal with structure, process and outcomes in these areas. Recommendations have been made about how the standards can be audited.

Retrospective Views of Bereaved Relatives
The Regional Study for the Care of the Dying used a well-tried methodology of interviewing relatives of patients who died of cancer. This approach permits comparison of different palliative-care and conventional-care services. However, the semi-structured interview is long and requires the expense of trained interviewers to administer it. The methodology is being adapted to a written questionnaire format which can be sent in the mail. This is similar to the Mortality Feed-back Survey which is conducted by mail in the United States.

Palliative-Care Assessment (PACA) Tool
This was developed by a hospital-based advisory palliative-care team. It includes items on symptoms, emotional status, social and patient-insight issues. PACA is scored by a health-care professional with the patient. After trials of validity and reliability, it has been used in hospice in-patient units, specialist home-care teams and district nursing services.

Patient Evaluated Problem Score (PEPS)
The PEPS has been recently developed for routine clinical use in hospice patients. The items are defined by the patient. The simple format allows the majority of patients to complete assessments up to the last 14 days of life, even into the last week of life. It has not been validated but the concept is an important new direction in instrument design.

Summary

One of the aims of palliative care is to maximise the quality of life experienced by terminally ill patients with cancer. Quality of life is a complex construct, reflecting physical, psychological, social, spiritual and other issues. Several questionnaires have been designed to measure various aspects of quality of life. Some of these instruments have been used to evaluate palliative-care services but there have been significant methodological problems. Most of the studies have shown that specialist palliative-care services are more effective than conventional care in relieving pain, improving satisfaction with care and supporting families. These benefits are associated with lower costs, particularly when palliative-care services are subsidised by charitable donations. Audit strategies have been devised which can help palliative-care services maintain the quality of their services.

11 – Ethical Issues and Palliative Care

Introduction

The care of terminally ill patients and families can raise some difficult ethical dilemmas. There are dilemmas about whether to start or stop 'active' anti-cancer treatments. Palliative care is directed at symptom control; what if the patient refuses to take medications to relieve symptoms? What happens if a patient wants to die at home but the family refuses to care for the patient? What about euthanasia? These, and other, problems are constantly presenting themselves to palliative-care practitioners. Because the emotional atmosphere is already charged when caring for the terminally ill, it is important to understand the ethical issues before they are confronted.

Ethical Issues in Palliative Care

Traditionally, doctors have made decisions on behalf of patients. Doctors were considered to 'know what was best' by virtue of their medical training. Patients were thought to be incapable of understanding and participating in the decision-making process. At the turn of the century, the St Bartholomew's Hospital rules stated that 'every patient must strictly obey the Directions of the Physician or Surgeon under whose care he or she may be placed'. Any patients who failed to comply risked being 'admonished or discharged'. Such a paternalistic approach is no longer tenable in modern society. People have much higher expectations because they are better educated and informed. There is a constant stream of articles and reports on health-care issues in the media and on the World Wide Web. Cancer information services provide information by a variety of means, including telephone and booklets.

The ethical basis of medical decision-making has been re-examined in the light of these changes in public attitude. Beauchamp and Childress (1989) identified four key principles, as follows.

Patient Autonomy

The principle of autonomy affirms the right of the patient to determine how he or she will be treated. Patient choice is central to the decision-making process. In

order to make an informed choice, patients should be given sufficient information about the treatment options, time to ask questions and the freedom to
refuse treatment. Making decisions on behalf of a patient, without their consent,
is only ethically justified when they are not capable of understanding or making
decisions. One cannot label patients as incompetent just because they are not co-
operative and refuse treatment. However, patients who are confused, psychotic,
demented or comatose when dying may be unable to comprehend or decide.
Severely depressed patients may also have difficulty making decisions.

Beneficence

Beneficence is the principle of considering and offering treatments which are
likely to provide relief. Beneficence also includes the concepts of preventing
harm to patients or removing harm from them.

Non-Maleficence

Non-maleficence is the opposite of beneficence and entails not deliberately
setting out to harm the patient.

Justice

The principle of justice is extremely important. Justice has two aspects: absolute
and comparative. Absolute justice requires that issues which are not relevant to
the decision-making process should not be considered, for example, race, socio-
economic status and sexual orientation. Comparative justice holds that patient
choice is not absolute. For example, a patient may wish to have euthanasia but
this does not override the doctor's moral and legal obligation not to comply.
Comparative justice also takes the availability of resources into account. If
health-care resources are scarce, individual treatment options may have to take
the broader social consequences into account. A very expensive anti-cancer
treatment may not be made available because it would divert funds from cheaper
treatments that would benefit a larger number of patients. A potentially difficult
example involving comparative justice is the balance between a patient's desire
to be cared for at home and the reluctance of the spouse to care for the patient at
home.

Ethical Principles and Clinical Decision Making

In palliative care, as in any branch of medicine, these ethical principles must be
applied whenever a decision must be made about a clinical problem. In practice,
this involves the following issues.

Clearly Identifying the Problem

This involves listening to the patient and checking that you have understood what the problem is. The interview should take place in a quiet environment. There should be sufficient time to tailor the interview to the condition of the patient. Terminally ill patients are usually very weak and it is important to watch for exhaustion. It is better to begin with open-ended questions such as 'How is it affecting you?', letting the patient determine what 'it' is. When the patient has described his needs, more direct questions may be used to clarify specific points or to ask about symptoms which the patient has not mentioned, always trying not to put words in the patient's mouth. The patient usually has some ideas about what should be done for the problem and these should be explored. In some cases, patients who are showing signs of distress will ignore or deny distress from symptoms. Rather than press for acknowledgement of the apparent problem, it is better to demonstrate a commitment to the patient's wishes by allowing him to maintain a sense of control.

Advisory palliative-care teams must be particularly careful to understand what patients perceive to be their problems. These teams rely on referrals from other health-care professionals. Team members will soon learn that hospital staff may present problems such as pain when it is actually the staff who are having difficulty coping with the patient. Another common example is the patient who is tachypnoeic which is interpreted as breathlessness by the carers. However, symptoms which are by definition subjective experiences of the patient, should not be confused with signs.

It can be helpful interviewing relatives. They may provide valuable information about symptoms or psycho-social difficulties. It may be possible to find out about past experiences of cancer which may have a bearing on how the patient perceives his problems or how he interprets what is happening. Such information should not override the patient's perceptions.

Identifying the Options for Treating the Problem

As problems are defined, possible solutions can be devised. The team should have a forum for discussing strategies to address patient and family problems. Team meetings concentrate the variety of disciplines and individual talents of the members. Problem definition is greatly enhanced and several perspectives can be generated. Non-medical health-care professionals bring their own professional skills. With experience and encouragement, they can also contribute to the medical debate. This counters some of the inadequacies of the traditional medical model. Patients find it difficult to tell doctors about their concerns. They will often communicate their worries about treatment decisions with non-medical staff.

In general, several options should be presented. A range of possibilities will confirm that the patient's situation is being taken seriously and it also engenders a sense of security in the future. If the patient has expressed a clear choice already, this should be respected. Treatment options should be presented as an outline of what the treatment entails, what the potential risks and benefits are, and what the consequences of not choosing the treatment will be. The information should be recorded on tape or written down. Patients and families often need time to consider the implications and ask further questions. Relatives should be included in the process if the patient wishes.

If a problem requires urgent treatment, for example, the sudden onset of breathlessness with a chest infection, many patients recognise the need to make a quick decision. Usually they defer the decision to the doctor because they are feeling so ill or frightened. However, time should always be made available to review the decision as the patient's condition improves.

Some problems lie outside the collective experience of the team, such as an agitated depression or psychosis that may need psychiatric consultation. The team should recognise these limitations and not be afraid to seek the advice of others.

The team should then endeavour to support the patient's choice, but should remember that patients may change their views with time. While a patient may initially agree to a particular treatment, later non-compliance should be recognised as a choice, not as being 'unreasonable' or 'ungrateful'. Some patients acquiesce with a decision and then fail to comply with the treatment. This should not be interpreted as a personal affront by the doctor. Rather, it should prompt a careful review with the patient. It is better to make allowances for changes in patient choice by reviewing the treatment decisions at periodic intervals.

Occasionally, a patient will request a second opinion. As with non-compliance, this should not be interpreted as a slight on the doctor's judgement. The request should always be honoured with good grace. It can be helpful to offer a second opinion if the patient has indicated a preference for options which the team is familiar with or comfortable with. Paradoxically, such an offer will strengthen the relationship between the patient and the team. Patients usually interpret the offer as reassuring and affirming, rather than a sign of weakness or incompetence.

There are instances when a problem remains unsolved and all possibilities have been exhausted. In other cases, the problem may never be resolvable. In these situations, patients, family and staff will still benefit from ongoing support. Team members are likely to become worn down by frustration and disappointment and they need to share the load, especially if the illness is protracted.

Decision-Making for Hospital-Based Advisory Teams

The decision-making process is potentially fraught when the team does not have the primary responsibility for the care of the patient. In practice, it may be extremely difficult to present alternatives to the patient, particularly when the primary team is not willing or likely to fulfil the patient's choice. In some circumstances, a patient will be referred because he wants more treatment than the primary team are prepared to give. The expectation of the primary team will be that the palliative-care team member will persuade the patient to accept their decision. These problems become less likely with time, as the primary team becomes more confident with the skills and abilities of the palliative-care team.

In the hospital situation, there is a risk that the patient could become a battlefield between the 'care-oriented' palliative-care team and the 'cure-oriented' hospital teams. Maintaining the precedence of informed patient choice can be very difficult, particularly if the palliative-care team members subscribe to a philosophy that minimises active treatment. However, patients may well accept a considerable degree of risk from toxic treatments which hold minimal chances of benefit. These patients will quickly dismiss the efforts of a palliative-care team that is not comfortable with this choice.

Whenever patients have problems beyond the expertise of the team, it can be particularly helpful to discuss these with the local hospice, or a major teaching hospice. Very often, there will be staff within the hospital who can also help, but team members may be reluctant to ask for fear of appearing incompetent. However, staff often appreciate the chance to be involved and this will make them feel more comfortable about using the team. Even if the advice is not totally appropriate, the profile of the terminally ill will be raised. Joint collaboration will improve the mutual awareness of the options that are available to cancer patients. Palliative-care practitioners may underestimate the value of anti-cancer treatments and overestimate the side-effects. Conversely, cancer specialists may be unaware of specific symptom control measures that provide good palliation, for example, the medical management of malignant bowel obstruction.

Patient Competence to Make Decisions

Problems arise when a patient is not competent to make a decision. This occurs when a patient cannot take in information, process the information and then provide a response. Sometimes a patient cannot take in information because of the shock of the diagnosis, because of deafness, or because of language difficulties. In these situations, the patient's failure to 'understand' information does not constitute incompetence. Every effort must be made to recognise and overcome these problems. There are several situations in palliative care when incompetence may arise: depression, delirium and altered states of consciousness.

Clinical depression can cause patients to make decisions which they would not otherwise make if they were not depressed, such as the decision to commit suicide. Differentiating sadness from depression can be difficult in patients with symptoms of advanced cancer. Feelings of sadness are very common with the impending loss of future prospects, family relationships, etc. The vegetative physical symptoms of depression are also common: lethargy, loss of libido and loss of appetite. Other diagnostic markers must be considered, such as lack of self-worth. An expert psychiatric opinion may be needed.

Confusion is a common problem in the terminally ill. It may be due to reversible causes or may be part of the dying process. At times, this distinction is easily made. However, some reversible causes of confusion may mimic the signs of dying, for example, the effects of hypercalcaemia. If the patient has not previously expressed wishes about treatment in these cases, the reversible cause should be treated and decision confirmed when the patient recovers. When the patient is dying, the decision to relieve the confusion by sedating the patient should be taken by the doctor on behalf of the patient.

Involving the Family in Patient Treatment Decisions

Patients often want their spouses or close family to be involved in the decision-making process, at least to be aware of the treatment options. This is not always the case. If a patient wants information withheld from carers, this wish must be respected. The implications of the decision can be discussed with the patient. Any inclination to tell relatives about diagnosis and prognosis before telling the patient must be resisted. This can lead to a collusion between the family and doctor to 'protect' the patient. However, it only leads to severe disruption of relationships between all parties. Furthermore, the patient will be more distressed than if he or she had been informed.

When the patient and family are involved together, the patient's decision will often reflect a consensus opinion. Individual family members may disagree but will usually feel bound to collaborate to avoid upsetting the patient. Time should be made to allow the spouse to express concerns and doubts. It is always helpful to tell the patient that you are having such a meeting. Sometimes, the patient will be trying to protect the relative and vice versa. Opening up communication may help to reach a decision that is more beneficial to patient and family. If the patient remains set on a particular course of action, the relative will benefit from ongoing support.

Problems can arise when the patient's choice is diametrically opposed to the relative's choice, but the relative is needed to carry out the patient's decision. This commonly occurs when the patient wants to go home but the spouse cannot cope. If the patient has been the dominant partner in the relationship, the spouse will be made to feel guilty. Another example occurs when family decide not to care for a patient as a reaction to a life-long pattern of dysfunctional relationships with the patient. This leaves the patient feeling angry, rejected and abandoned. These situations are very stressful for staff as well. If the patient deteriorates quickly, place of care may not be such an issue when the patient becomes very weak in the terminal phase. However, some patients may live for many months, for example, with paraplegia from spinal cord compression. When these patients are cared for in a hospice, nursing teams may have to rotate the care to cope with the emotional load from the angry patient.

When the patient is not competent to make a decision, family members should be involved in discussions about treatment. This is especially important in the acute hospital setting where relatives are too reticent to ask staff questions for fear of interrupting the busy ward schedule. Involvement of the family in a decision to withdraw or withhold 'active' treatment must be done carefully. They should not be made to feel responsible for the decision. This can leave them feeling guilty and responsible for the patient's death. Furthermore, relatives will often include their own needs in the decision, for example, to keep the patient alive at any cost. The family should be asked if the patient ever expressed any wishes about what he or she would have wanted done. They should also be asked for their feelings about what should be done. The final decision should then be taken by the physician in charge, taking into account the stated aims of the patient if these are known, the feelings of the family and staff, and the expected risks:benefits of the treatments given the clinical context. If the decision is different from the wishes of the family, time will be needed for careful explanation and support.

Occasionally, the family may strongly disagree with the physician's decision. In these circumstances, it may be possible to come to some compromise that does not increase the suffering of the patient. For example, the withholding of intravenous rehydration in dying patients often worries families. Unfortunately, some palliative-care physicians argue from a philosophical standpoint that patients should be allowed to die with dignity and that intravenous rehydration is undignified. This can potentially inflame conflict if the family has a different philosophy. Rather than base the discussion on philosophical principles, a simple explanation of the altered physiology of fluid balance in the terminally ill is usually sufficient to put the family's minds at rest. If not, some level of compromise should be possible as long as the patient had not previously expressed a preference against rehydration. A low volume (500–1000 ml/day) infusion of normal saline subcutaneously will avoid the effects of fluid overload, minimise discomfort to the patient and assuage the concerns of the family.

Quality of Life and Medical Decision-Making

The issue of quality of life often features in decision-making. Some palliative-care practitioners have the goal of maximising quality of life, which means controlling symptoms, getting the patient to accept death, and minimising 'active' treatments. On the other hand, acute hospital doctors will decide that a certain treatment should not be offered because the patient's quality of life is perceived as being too poor. This usually means that the doctors cannot see that they would have any quality of life if they were as ill as the patient. Both of these perspectives suffer from the fact that they are imposed on patients.

Quality of life is a subjective experience and only the patient can or should make judgements about it. Patients protect themselves psychologically from the full impact of a terminal disease. Relatives and health-care professionals tend to overrate patients' symptoms and underrate patients' satisfaction with life. This is partly due to carers loading their own anxieties and sense of helplessness into their judgements about the patients.

Patients make trade-offs between quantity and quality of life. Slevin et al. (1990) found that patients were prepared to accept a cure rate from chemotherapy as low as 1%, even though the treatment could be very toxic. Some patients prefer to avoid any anti-cancer treatments, opting for quality rather than extended life. Most people want to maximise both. This is one of the most compelling reasons for a closer collaboration between palliative and acute cancer care.

Resource Allocation and Patient Choice

All Western economies are facing a crisis in health-care funding. Costs of investigations and treatments are escalating dramatically. The expectations of patients and families are also increasing. However, economic reality means that implicit health-care rationing exists, for example, in the form of 'waiting lists'. The likelihood is that the relative expenditure on health care will fall, further reducing treatment options. The idea of explicit rationing is being considered more widely. Politically, it is not expedient to openly categorise treatment availability. Inevitably, however, some treatments will cease to be available or will be very difficult to access.

Ethical Dilemmas in Palliative Care

There are a number of ethical problems which arise when treating terminally ill patients. This section reviews the issues of sedation and symptom control, euthanasia, and fluid replacement therapy for the dying.

Sedation and Symptom Control

One of the key aims of symptom control is to relieve symptoms and maximise quality of life. When medications are used, there is always a potential trade-off between side-effects and benefits. Drowsiness is a side-effect of several drugs used in palliative care, a side-effect which most patients dislike. Careful titration of medications against the symptom will minimise drowsiness. An example was described in the section on using morphine for pain control (page 24). Using these techniques should ensure that over 90% of patients should have minimal or no pain.

What about the rare occasions when pain is not controlled? It is always possible to increase the dose of centrally acting analgesics such as morphine until the pain is controlled, but this may produce sedation. If the sedation is severe enough, the patient will develop a pneumonia and die. The medication will successfully relieve the physical distress but will cause death to occur before the expected effects of the cancer. The ethical dilemma is whether to relieve the patient's symptom but in so doing hasten death, or to leave the patient in distress. Medical and theological ethicists agree that the first priority must be to relieve suffering, even though this may hasten death. This is known as the principle of the double-effect. Double-effect is distinguished from euthanasia by the intention behind the treatment. With the former, the primary intention is to relieve suffering recognising that death may follow; the primary intention of euthanasia is to kill the patient to relieve the suffering.

The sedation of very agitated and confused patients is another example of a clinical situation which evokes the principle of double-effect. Some patients may still have lucid intervals which they enjoy despite being confused most of the time. However, patients who are continually distressed require regular medication. Rigorous efforts to relieve agitation but avoid sedation usually fail; the patient is only settled when sedated. A decision then has to be taken to continue regular sedation so that the patient remains asleep for long periods of time. This increases the risk of the patient developing a pneumonia and dying more quickly. The primary intent of treatment, however, is to relieve the patient's distress, not to kill the patient.

Although the principle of double-effect satisfies the ethical demands of these rare clinical scenarios, it can be difficult to explain to distressed relatives, upset by what they see as killing the patient. A careful explanation of the medical issues is needed. The common theme with these patients is their weakened cachectic physical state owing to the effects of advanced cancer. In the absence of severe pain or agitation, these patients would normally be drowsy and lying in bed feeling too weak to move. However, the excitatory, rather than the depressant, pathways in the brain have been released from control, which is why the distress will rapidly escalate and become extreme if treatment is not given. Relief of the distress allows the patient to return to the normal physical state of a dying patient, hence the reason why a balance between symptom relief without sedation cannot be achieved with careful titration.

Euthanasia

Euthanasia literally means 'good death'. In this section, euthanasia will be defined as the deliberate killing of a terminally ill patient by administration of a lethal substance, usually given by injection. This practice is currently illegal in the United Kingdom. The term 'passive' euthanasia is sometimes used to describe the withholding of life-prolonging treatments such as artificial ventilation for patients who are brain-dead. This process is sanctioned ethically and legally in appropriate circumstances. It should not be described as euthanasia; this has been a major source of confusion in the euthanasia debate.

Proponents of euthanasia originally argued that 'mercy-killing' was necessary as a last resort for treating unrelieved suffering. The modern hospice movement has clearly demonstrated that suffering can always be relieved and that no patient need die in agony. The recent House of Lords Commission on Medical Ethics (Walton, 1994), which was convened in England to review the law about euthanasia, agreed with this conclusion. The report argued that legalisation of euthanasia was not an option. It recommended that palliative-care services should be made more widely available. These findings have shifted the debate on to the following two issues.

Relieving Symptoms Using the Double-Effect is the Same as Euthanasia Anyway

Recent studies of the attitudes and practices of doctors are quoted in support of the idea that euthanasia is practised anyway, so why not legalise it? A study of general practitioners (Ward and Tate, 1994) is cited as evidence, with at least one-third of GPs believing they have practised euthanasia. Careful analysis of the study reveals that less than 10% of the doctors surveyed gave this response. The exact way in which those doctors administered euthanasia is not described. However, many doctors still believe that giving injections of morphine to terminally ill patients is tantamount to euthanasia. This only serves to emphasise the need for more education in palliative care and better access to hospice services, rather than liberalising euthanasia.

Individual Patients Should Have the Right to Choose to Have Their Lives Ended Consistent with the Principle of Patient Autonomy

The current legal situation is held up as an example of infringement of personal freedom. The practice of allowing euthanasia in Holland, even though it has not been legalised, is cited as an example of good practice. The state of Oregon in the USA and the Northern Territories in Australia have considered legislation to condone euthanasia performed by doctors – so-called 'physician-assisted suicide'. Safeguards have been introduced to prevent abuses of the law. More than one doctor is required to certify that the patient is competent and has made an informed choice for euthanasia. An appropriate time interval, usually weeks, is required before the patient confirms the choice, then euthanasia is performed.

Holland is the only country where the effects of liberalising access to euthanasia can be assessed. Official statistics have been kept on the number of cases and the reasons for euthanasia. An analysis of these statistics reveals some disturbing trends. The number of reported cases is relatively low, only 2% of the total number of cancer deaths. However, in many cases the permission of the patient was not sought or could not be obtained. This is called involuntary euthanasia and sets a dangerous precedent, doctors making judgements about euthanasia on behalf of patients. The discrepancy between doctors' and patients' interpretations of quality of life has already been described in this chapter. Allowing doctors to make quality-of-life decisions which might lead to euthanasia places the vulnerable in society at grave risk: the elderly, mentally infirm and physically handicapped. There have already been widely publicised cases, one where a doctor killed a physically deformed infant, another where a depressed woman who felt that life was not worth living was given euthanasia. Even more worrying is the evidence that the aforementioned safeguards do not protect against abuse of the law. There is now disturbing evidence that at least as many patients are given euthanasia but are not reported officially (Van der Wal and Dillmann, 1994). These are all signs of the 'slippery slope' phenomenon, where a steady slide is occurring towards even more liberal interpretations of euthanasia which are already affecting the vulnerable. The responsibility of society is to protect the weak. This must take precedence over the rights of the individual. Patient autonomy must be balanced by comparative social justice.

A factor which is often overlooked in promoting the Dutch experience is the paucity of palliative-care services in Holland (Zylicz, 1993). There are very few hospices. Holland has one of the lowest per capita uses of oral morphine in Europe, despite having some of the most liberal opioid prescribing laws. A recent BBC television documentary portrayed the actual killing of a patient with motor neurone disease. The doctor told the patient and his wife that death would be distressing, that he would suffocate or drown at the end. Not surprisingly, the patient opted for euthanasia given this prospect. However, patients with motor neurone disease do not choke to death (O'Brien et al., 1992). The patient was misinformed, which only emphasises the need for better palliative care. It is of interest that the Northern Territories is the only part of Australia with virtually no specialist palliative-care services.

In conclusion, euthanasia should not be made legal. There is no need for patients to die in agony if palliative care is available. Legalising euthanasia exposes the vulnerable in society to 'mercy-killing'. This cannot be prevented by stringent safeguards.

Handling a Patient Who Requests Euthanasia

It is perhaps surprising that so few patients ask for euthanasia, even in situations where the option is condoned. This testifies to the resilience of the human spirit, even in situations which seem hopeless. However, there are occasions when a patient will say that death would be preferable; some even ask outright for euthanasia. It is important to know how to respond when this happens. Usually, the patient makes a comment rather than a request. Even so, the response must be measured. Some health-care professionals feel so strongly against euthanasia that they launch into a diatribe against it, which by implication makes the patient feel culpable. This reaction is totally unacceptable. More commonly, health-care professionals sense the anguish behind the patient's statement but they try to encourage the patient to feel more hopeful: 'things can't be that bad' or 'cheer up, think of your family', are examples. Such comments only serve to increase the patient's sense of isolation.

The best approach is to acknowledge the patient's feelings as valid, regardless of the legal or moral status of euthanasia. The patient should be encouraged to talk about why these feelings have arisen and what the fears about the future are. A direct request for euthanasia should be met with an affirmation of the patient's integrity and motivation for asking, followed by an unambiguous statement that the request cannot be fulfilled. Patients will respect a direct and honest response. Health-care professionals should avoid confusing the discussion by exposing their personal doubts to the patient. Most patients are relieved at the chance to air their concerns and are reassured by the prospect of ongoing support. When anguish persists, the strategies outlined in the chapter on spiritual pain are needed.

Nutrition and Fluid Replacement Therapy for Dying Patients

Terminally ill cancer patients experience increasing anorexia. Eventually, most patients stop eating and then stop drinking. The management of weight loss and poor appetite was discussed in Chapter 5. Even with the use of drugs like steroids, there comes a time when these options are not effective. Craig (1994) has drawn attention to the dilemma which then arises: whether or not to give dying patients nutritional support and fluid replacement therapy. Hospices do not routinely give intravenous fluids in the terminal phase. With normal people, this would cause starvation and dehydration. If dehydration is not treated quickly, the person becomes very symptomatic, deteriorates rapidly and death quickly follows. How should the situation be managed with a patient who is already dying?

The first important clinical judgement is to distinguish between a dying patient who is not drinking and a patient with advanced cancer who is not dying but has become dehydrated. In the latter case, the patient's condition will have been relatively stable and then suddenly have deteriorated. Other causes of the decline will be evident, such as hypercalcaemia or infection. These causes may precipitate dehydration as a secondary effect, with clinical signs of low blood volume and biochemical evidence of renal impairment and electrolyte disturbance. If the secondary dehydration is not treated, the patient will die of the consequences. These patients should receive a trial of intravenous fluid replacement unless they have expressly requested otherwise.

Patients who has been deteriorating more slowly from the general effects of advanced cancer will spontaneously give up drinking. They will often appreciate being given small amounts of ice to suck or other simple measures to keep the mouth moist. However, they do not ask for and may even refuse fluids to drink. The usual signs of dehydration, such as dry mouth and excessive thirst, are not present. If the patient is able to make a decision and does not want to drink, this should be honoured. Sometimes the patient will try to drink fluids to avoid distressing the carers. This can cause aspiration and coughing bouts which are even more troubling to the patient. The family should be gently dissuaded. Their concern to care should be redirected to moistening the lips or offering pieces of ice.

The ethical dilemma is brought sharply into focus when, as is usually the case, patients are too ill and too drowsy to make their wishes known. The decision about nutritional and fluid support falls to the staff and family. Eating and drinking are so fundamental to life that when the patient stops, the certainty of death cannot be denied. This realisation can be distressing enough but strong religious and cultural demands may require that the patient be nourished until the end to avoid any sense of blame for causing the death.

Any clinical decision must be based on a clear understanding of the risks and benefits of treatments versus no treatment. This is even more important when the clinical situation is very emotionally charged as well. The medical value of nutritional support is highly questionable. Conventional intravenous fluids containing dextrose are appropriate for fluid replacement only. The caloric value of dextrose even in the 5% solutions is minimal and not sufficient to prevent malnutrition. Normal daily requirements can only be met with high concentrations of dextrose given with amino acids, lipids and essential vitamins, etc. Even if this is given intravenously into a central vein, there is no evidence that parenteral nutrition causes the patient to live any longer. Although dying patients appear to be malnourished, the metabolic abnormalities are quite different, hence the lack of effectiveness. There is some evidence that cancer growth is accelerated. Given the lack of benefit, there is no justification for nutritional support in dying cancer patients.

The effects of not giving fluid replacement have been studied in patients dying from cancer. Electrolyte disturbances are not common. Even when there is biochemical evidence of dehydration, there is no significant increase in symptoms such as dry mouth and thirst, at least in those patients who are still able to communicate (Ellershaw et al., 1995). In these patients, dry mouth is much more likely to be due to drugs such as hyoscine. It would seem that the normal fluid balance, and therefore fluid requirements, may be different in patients who are dying. Fluid replacement therapy seems to offer no benefit. Waller et al. (1991) reported that intravenous fluids did not improve the clinical or the biochemical status of dying patients with biochemical evidence of dehydration and altered consciousness.

There are risks to giving 'replacement' fluids, whether by intravenous or subcutaneous routes. Dying patients often have lower levels of serum albumin. Even 'normal' volumes of fluids cannot be held in the intravascular compartment because of lowered oncotic pressure. This increases peripheral oedema. The legs can become swollen and uncomfortable, the hands and subconjunctival tissues become puffy and unsightly. Dyspnoea can be made worse and pulmonary oedema may even occur.

Based on the risks and lack of demonstrable benefit, the routine use of fluid replacement therapy cannot be justified medically. In practice, a few families will not be reassured by a careful explanation of these observations. They remain distressed at the thought that they may be morally responsible for the patient's death. Sometimes, a spiritual advisor will reassure them that theological concerns are not warranted. For example, some Roman Catholic families still believe that the Church demands that anything less than fluid therapy given right up to the moment when the patient dies will be euthanasia. Even so, there are rare situations where the distress of the relatives cannot be assuaged. Then, provided the patient has not given clear instructions to the contrary, a small volume of fluid can be given. No more than one litre of fluid can be given subcutaneously per day with no distress to the patient, but considerable relief to the family.

The Patient Who Refuses Symptom Control

The relief of distressing symptoms such as pain is central to the practice of palliative care. Most patients are only too grateful to be made comfortable. Patients who refuse to take analgesics, or any treatment which staff feel will make them appear less distressed, cause pain for the carers. Nurses find it very stressful looking after patients who refuse physical cares. Dying patients are physically weak and often feel vulnerable. It is possible to persuade patients to take medications in the hospice setting because they worry about offending the carers. At home, the patient is more likely to hold out against advice, causing more stress to the relatives as well.

The ethical principle of autonomy requires that the patient's decision not to take advice or medications should be respected. It may help to realise that the patient will suffer more from the psychological distress of having to take medication than from the symptom. This should prompt a discussion with the patient about why the prospect of treatment is so worrying. The timing of such a discussion is important. Too early in the relationship and the patient will feel under pressure, not respected. It is often better to support the patient's decision for the first few visits until trust is established. If the patient is denying the symptom, it is better not to try and break this down. Establishing a rapport will be difficult if the uncontrolled symptom is maintained as the focus. It is often more helpful to find out what you can do that the patient will perceive as helpful.

Sometimes, the patient's judgement will be based on deeply held misinformation, such as the fear of addiction or early death from morphine. Gently correcting this may allow the patient to make a more informed choice. Having supported the patient's initial choice, the information from the health-care professional will be less threatening and more readily received. Significant past experiences, such as the prior death of a parent or friend, may be an important cause of the patient's fears. Here again, trust is needed to reveal and perhaps reduce the impact of these experiences.

Some patients persist in their denial. The health-care professionals must remain committed to the long process of sincerely trying to understand and respect the patient's views of the illness and treatment. These views may seem quite bizarre. For example, a man with lung cancer was frightened that any medication would explode inside his chest. He was not mentally ill or confused. Any attempt to override his concerns caused extreme distress, much worse than his breathlessness. By understanding his reasoning, it was possible to appreciate why he would not take medication. It was not possible or appropriate to persist in trying to change a deeply entrenched construct, no matter how unusual.

Whenever this situation arises, the professional team will need to support each other if they are to support the patient. The team may also need to support the relatives if they do not share the patient's view. The helplessness of relatives can be reduced if they can off-load their frustrations. The professional team will need to remind themselves, and the relatives, that the patient's ability to tolerate symptoms will diminish rapidly when the patient begins to die. Then, the symptom will escalate and cause extreme distress. If this happens, the patient will often want treatment and will trust the judgement of the professionals because they have respected the wishes, and therefore the dignity, of the patient.

Conclusion

Palliative care is a new specialty which has advanced quickly in the 30 years since the founding of St Christopher's Hospice. The holistic approach which addresses physical, psychological, social and spiritual needs of patients and families has bought new hope when previously doctors felt that nothing more could be done. The challenges for palliative care are to find new and better options for patients and families, to demonstrate the effectiveness of the palliative-care approach, and to educate other health-care professionals in the skills of palliative care. The ultimate challenge is to weave the palliative-care approach so closely into the fabric of health care that all aspects of health care are affected, not just the care of people with advanced cancer.

References

Aaronson NK, Ahmedzai S, Bergman B, et al. (1993). The European Organisation for Research and Treatment of Cancer QLQ-C30: a quality of life instrument for use in international clinical trials in oncology. Journal of the National Cancer Institute, 85: 365–376.

Addington-Hall J, McCarthy M (1995). Regional study of care for the dying: methods and sample characteristics. Palliative Medicine, 9: 27–36.

Ashby MA, Game PA, Davit P, Britten-Jones R, Brooksbank MA, Davy MLJ and Keam E (1991). Percutaneous gastrostomy as a venting procedure in palliative care. Palliative Medicine, 5(2): 147–150.

Baines M (1993). The pathophysiology and management of malignant intestinal obstruction. Oxford Textbook of Palliative Medicine, OUP, Oxford, pp. 311–316.

Baines MJ, Oliver DJ, and Carter RL (1985). Medical management of intestinal obstruction in patients with advanced malignant disease: a clinical and pathological study. Lancet, ii: 990–993.

Beattie GJ, Leonard RCF and Smyth JF (1989). Bowel obstruction in ovarian cancer: a retrospective study and review of the literature. Palliative Medicine, 3: 275–280.

Beauchamp TL, Childress JF (1989). Principles of Biomedical Ethics. OUP, Oxford, 3rd edn.

Bergner M, Bobbitt RA, Carter WB et al. (1981). The sickness impact profile: development and final revision of a health status measure. Medical Care, 19: 787–805.

Bruera E, Higginson I (Eds) (1996). Cachexia–Anorexia in Cancer Patients. OUP, Oxford.

Carter RL, Pittam MR, Tanner NSB (1982). Pain and dysphagia in patients with squamous carcinomas of the head and neck: the role of perineural spread. Journal of the Royal Society of Medicine, 75: 598–606.

Cassell EJ (1982). The nature of suffering and the goals of medicine. New England Journal of Medicine, 306: 639–645.

Cleeland CS, Gonin R, Hatfield AK et al. (1994). Pain and pain treatment in outpatients with metastatic cancer: the Eastern Co-operative Oncology Group's Out-patient Pain Study. New England Journal of Medicine, 331: 592–596.

Craig GM (1994). On withholding nutrition and hydration in the terminally ill: has palliative medicine gone too far? Journal of Medical Ethics, 20: 139–143.

Crosby P. (1976). Quality is Free. McGraw-Hill, New York.

Davis CL, Ahern R (1996). Single dose randomised controlled trial of nebulised morphine in patients with cancer-related breathlessness. Palliative Medicine, 10: 64–65.

Day RO, Brooks PM (1987). Variations in response to non-steroidal drugs. British Journal of Clinical Pharmacology, 23: 655–658.

De Haes JCJM, Van Knippenberg FCE, Neijt JP (1990). Measuring psychological and physical distress in cancer patients: structure and application of the Rotterdam Symptom Checklist. British Journal of Cancer, 62: 1034–1038.

De Wys WD, Begg C, Lavin PT et al. (1980). Prognostic effect of weight loss prior to chemotherapy in cancer patients. American Journal of Medicine, 69: 491–497.

Deschamps M, Band PR, Hyslop TG et al. (1992). The evaluation of analgesics in cancer patients as exemplified by a double-blind cross-over study of immediate release versus controlled release morphine. Journal of Pain and Symptom Management, 7: 384–392.

Dunlop RJ, Hockley JM, Davies RJ (1989). Preferred versus actual place of death – a hospital terminal care support team experience. Palliative Medicine, 3: 197–201.

Ellershaw JE, Sutcliffe J, Saunders CM (1995). Dehydration and the dying patient. Journal of Pain and Symptom Management, 10: 192–197.

Emanuel EJ (1996). Cost savings at the end of life: what do the data show? Journal of the American Medical Association, 275: 1907–1914.

Fainsinger RL, MacEachern T, Miller MJ, Bruera E, Spachynski K, KueLn N, Hanson J. (1994) The use of hypodermoclysis for rehydration in terminally ill cancer patients. The Journal of Pain and Symptom Management, 9: 298–302.

Ferrell BA (1991). Pain management in elderly people. Journal of the American Geriatric Society, 39: 64–73.

Fishman B, Pasternak S, Wallenstein SL et al. (1987). The Memorial Pain Assessment Chart: a valid instrument for the evaluation of cancer pain. Cancer, 60: 1151–1158.

Gemio B, Rayner AA, Lewis B (1986). Home support of patients with end-stage malignant bowel obstruction using hydration and venting gastrostomy. The American Journal of Surgery, 152: 100–104.

Grant M, Padilla GV, Ferrell BR et al. (1990). Assessment of quality of life with a single instrument. Seminars in Oncology Nursing, 6: 260–270.

Greer DS, Mor V, Kastenbaum R (Eds) (1988). The hospice experiment. Johns Hopkins Press, Baltimore.

Guadagnoli E, Mor V (1989). Measuring cancer patients' affect: revision and psychometric properties of the profile of mood states (POMS). Psychometric Assessments, 1: 150–154.

Heit HA, Johnson LF, Siegal SR, Boyce HW (1978). Palliative dilation for dysphagia in esophageal carcinoma. Annals of Internalal Medicine, 89: 629–631.

Herxheimer A, Begent R, MacLean D, et al. (1985). Short life of a terminal care support team: experience at Charing Cross Hospital. British Medical Journal, 290: 1877–1879.

Higginson I (Ed.) (1993). Clinical audit in palliative care. Radcliffe, Oxford.

Hill F, Oliver C. (1989). Hospice – an update on the cost of patient care. Palliative Medicine, 3: 119–124.

Hinton J. (1963). The physical and mental distress of the dying. Quarterly Journal of Medicine, 32: 1–21.

Hinton J. (1979). Comparison of places and policies for terminal care. Lancet, i: 29–32.

Hockley JM, Dunlop RJ, Davies RJ (1988). Survey of distressing symptoms in dying patients and their families in hospital and the response to a symptom control team. British Medical Journal, 296: 1715–1717.

Jensen DM, Machicado G, Randall G et al. (1988). Comparison of low power YAG laser and BICAP tumour probe for palliation of esophageal cancer strictures. Gastroenterology, 94: 1263–1270.

Johnson I, Patterson S. (1992). Drugs used in combination in the syringe driver – a survey of hospice practice. Palliative Medicine, 6:125–30

Jones RVH (1993). Teams and terminal cancer at home: do patients and carers benefit? Journal on Interprofessional Care, 7: 239–244.

Kane RL, Wales J, Bernstein L et al. (1984). A randomised controlled trial of hospice care. Lancet, i: 890–894.

Kastenbaum R (1988). Problems of death and dying. In: Gilmore A, Gilmore S (Eds), Safe Death, Plenum Press, New York, pp. 3–14.

Kinnunen O, Janhonen P, Salokannel J, Kivela SL (1989). Diarrhoea and faecal impaction in elderly long stay patients. Z. Gerontologie, 22: 321–323.

Kristjansen LJ (1986). Indicators of quality of palliative care from a family perspective. Journal of Palliative Care, 1: 8–17.

Linn MW, Linn BS, Harris R (1982). Effects of counselling for late stage cancer patients.

Cancer, 49: 1048–1055.

Loizou LA, Greigs D, Atkinson M et al. (1992). A prospective comparison of laser therapy and intubation in endoscopic palliation for malignant dysphagia. Gastroenterology, 100: 1303–1310.

MacAdam DB, Smith M (1987). An initial assessment of suffering in terminal illness. Palliative Medicine, 1: 37–47.

McCorkle R, Young K (1978). Development of a symptom distress scale. Cancer Nursing, 1: 373–378.

Malone JM, Koonce T, Larson DM, Freedman RS, Carrasco CHO and Saul PB (1986). Palliation of small bowel obstruction by percutaneous gastrostomy in patients with progressive ovarian carcinoma. Obstetrics and Gynecology, 68: 431–433.

Mercadante S, Spoldi E, Caraceni A, Maddaloni S, Simonetti MT (1993). Octreotide in relieving gastrointestinal symptoms due to bowel obstruction. Palliative Medicine, 7: 295–299.

Moore N (1918). The history of St Bartholomew's Hospital, Pearson, London.

Mor V (1986). Assessing patient outcomes in a hospice: what to measure? In: Psychosocial Assessment in Terminal Care. Haworth Press, New York, 17–35.

Mor V, Masterton-Allen S (1987). Hospice care systems: structure, process, costs and outcome. Springer-Verlag, New York.

Mount BM, Jones A, Patterson A (1974). Death and dying: attitudes in a teaching hospital. Urology, 4: 741–747.

Mount BM, Scott JF (1983). Whither hospice evaluation? Journal of Chronic Diseases, 36: 731–736.

Mumford SP (1986). Can high fibre diets improve the bowel function in patients on a radiotherapy ward? Cited in: Twycross RG, Lack SA (Eds.) Control of Alimentary Symptoms in Far Advanced Cancer. Churchill Livingstone, London, 166–207.

Muurinen JM (1986). The economics of informal care: labour market effects in the National Hospice Study. Medical Care, 24: 1007–1017.

National Council for Hospice and Specialist Palliative Care Services (1995). Opening doors: improving access to hospice and specialist palliative care services by members of the black and ethnic minority community. National Hospice Council for Hospice and Specialist Palliative Care Services, London.

O'Brien T, Kelly M, Saunders CM (1992). Motor neurone disease: a hospice perspective. British Medical Journal, 304: 471–473.

Padilla GV, Ferrell B, Grant M, et al. (1990). Defining the content domain of quality of life for cancer patients with pain. Cancer Nursing, 13: 108–115.

Parkes, CM (1980). Bereavement counselling: does it work? British Medical Journal, 281: 3–6.

Parkes CM (1981). Evaluation of a bereavement service. Journal of Preventive Psychiatry, 1: 179–188.

Parkes CM (1997). Death and bereavement across cultures. Routledge, New York.

Parkes CM, Parkes J (1984). Hospice versus hospital care – re-evaluation after 10 years as seen by surviving spouses. Postgraduate Medical Journal, 60: 120–124.

Raphael B (1977). Preventive intervention with the recently bereaved. Archives of General Psychiatry, 34: 1450–1454.

Rice MI, Van Rij RIJ (1987). Parenteral nutrition and tumour growth in the patient with complicated abdominal cancer. Australia and New Zealand Journal of Surgery, 57: 375–379.

Riley J, Fallon MT (1994). Octreotide in terminal malignant obstruction of the gastro-intestinal tract. European Journal of Palliative Care, 1: 23–25.

Rowland CG, Pagliero KM (1985). Intracavitary irradiation in palliation of carcinoma of oesophagus and cardia. Lancet, ii: 981–983.

Schag CC, Heinrich RL, Ganz PA (1984). Karnofsky performance status revisited: reliability, validity and guidelines. Journal of Clinical Oncology, 12(3): 187–193.

Schipper H, Clinch J, McMurray A et al. (1984). Measuring the quality of life in cancer patients: the Functional Living Index – Cancer: development and validation. Journal of Clinical Oncology, 2: 472–483.

Schug SA, Zech D, Dorr U (1990). Cancer pain management according to WHO analgesic guidelines. Journal of Pain and Symptom Management, 5: 27–32.

Schug SA, Zech D, Grond S et al. (1992). A long-term survey of morphine in cancer pain patients. Journal of Pain and Symptom Management, 7: 259–266.

Seale CF (1991). A comparison of hospice and conventional care. Social Science and Medicine, 32: 147–152.

Seale CF, Cartwright A (1994). The year before death. Athenaeum Press, Newcastle.

Seale CF, Kelly M (1997). A comparison of hospice and hospital care for people who die: views of the surviving spouse. Palliative medicine, 11: 93–100.

Slevin ML, Stubbs L, Lynch D et al. (1990). Who should measure quality of life, the doctor or the patient? British Journal of Cancer, 300: 1458–1460.

Solomon S, Greenburg G, Pyszczynski T (1995). A terror management theory of social behaviour: the psychological functions of self-esteem and cultural world views. In: Zanna MP (Ed.), Advances in Experimental Social Psychology. Academic Press, San Diego, 91–159.

Steward AL, Hays RD, Ware JL (1988). The MOS short-form general health survey reliability and validity in a patient population. Medical Care, 26: 724–735.

Spitzer WO, Dobson AJ, Hall J et al. (1981). Measuring the quality of life of cancer patients: a concise QL index for use by physicians. Journal of Chronic Diseases, 34: 585–597.

Swerdlow M, Cundhill JG (1981). Anticonvulsant drugs used in the treatment of lancinating pain: a comparison. Anaesthesia, 36: 1129–1132.

Sykes NP, Baines MJ, Carter RL (1988). Clinical and pathological study of dysphagia conservatively managed in patients with advanced malignant disease. Lancet, ii: 726–728.

Vachon MLS (1987). Occupational stress in the care of the critically ill, the dying and the bereaved. Hemisphere, Washington.

Van der Wal G, Dillmann (1994). Euthanasia in the Netherlands. British Medical Journal, 308: 1346–1349.

Ventafridda V, Ripamonti C, Caraceni A, et al. (1990). The management of inoperable gastrointestinal obstruction in terminal cancer patients. Tumori, 76: 389–393.

Waller A, Adunski A, Hershkowitz M (1991). Terminal dehydration and intravenous fluids. Lancet, 337: 745.

Walton L (1994). Report of the Select Committee on Medical Ethics. HMSO, London.

Ward BJ, Tate PA (1994). Attitudes among NHS doctors to requests for euthanasia. British Medical Journal, 308: 1332–1334.

Wilkes E (1984). Dying now. Lancet, i: 950–952.

World Health Organization (1990). Cancer pain relief and palliative care. Technical Report Series 804. World Health Organization, Geneva.

Zigmond AS, Smith RP (1983). The Hospital Anxiety and Depression Scale. Acta Psychiatrica Scandinavia, 67: 361–370.

Zubrod CG, Schneiderman M, Frei E et al. (1960). Appraisal of methods for the study of chemotherapy of cancer in man: comparative therapeutic trial of nitrogen mustard and triethylene thiophosphoramide. Journal of Chronic Diseases, 11: 7–33.

Zylicz Z (1993). Hospice in Holland: the story behind the blank spot. American Journal of Hospice and Palliative Care, 10: 30–34.

Index